# THE PHYSIOLOGY AND BIOMECHANICS OF CYCLING

# AMERICAN COLLEGE OF SPORTS MEDICINE SERIES

**SKI CONDITIONING**
Merle Foss and James G. Garrick

**CONDITIONING FOR DISTANCE RUNNING:
THE SCIENTIFIC ASPECTS**
Jack Daniels, Robert Fitts, and George Sheehan

**THE PHYSIOLOGY AND BIOMECHANICS OF CYCLING**
Irvin Faria and Peter Cavanagh

**HEALTH AND FITNESS THROUGH
PHYSICAL ACTIVITY**
Michael Pollock, Jack Wilmore, and Samuel Fox

# THE PHYSIOLOGY AND BIOMECHANICS OF CYCLING

**IRVIN E. FARIA**
California State University,
Sacramento

**PETER R. CAVANAGH**
The Pennsylvania State
University

Cartoons by
ANN VANDERVELDE

JOHN WILEY & SONS
New York   Santa Barbara   Chichester   Brisbane   Toronto

*Library of Congress Cataloging in Publication data:*

Faria, Irvin.
    The physiology and biomechanics of cycling.

    1. Cycling–Physiological aspects. 2. Human mechanics. I. Cavanagh, Peter R., joint author.
    II. Title.
    RC1220. C8F38        612'.044        77-20245
    ISBN 0-471-25490-8

Printed in the United States of America

10  9  8  7  6  5  4  3  2  1

# FOREWORD

During the past 10 years, a tremendous explosion of knowledge has occurred in the exercise and sport sciences. New theories in the coaching and training of athletes have emerged, technological breakthroughs have allowed a better understanding of how people perform and adapt to the stress of exercise, and we now have a better understanding as to how exercise can improve both the quality and quantity of life. In addition, the population of the United States has become more conscious of physical fitness and has started exercising on their own, with little or no knowledge of what to do or how to go about it. Consequently, many commercial enterprises have evolved to satisfy this basic consumer need. Although many of these enterprises have provided valuable consumer services, there are many others that have not had the consumer's best interests at heart and have taken advantage of the general lack of knowledge of the average consumer.

In 1973, the American College of Sports Medicine, at the suggestion of their former President, Dr. Howard G. Knuttgen, planned a series of volumes to help bridge the widening gap between the latest research in the exercise and sport sciences and the consumer. The purpose of this Series was to bring to the level of the average consumer, the facts and basic information related to exercise in general, and individual sports specifically, in an interesting and unbiased manner. Dr. David L. Costill, currently President of the American College of Sports Medicine, was asked to initiate this Series.

v

The American College of Sports Medicine's Series is an exciting step forward in the area of consumer education. Each volume is co-authored by authorities in their respective areas, who were selected for their ability to communicate their ideas at a very practical and fundamental level. While each of these authors is a recognized scientist, each volume represents an attempt to apply the teachings and findings of science to the better understanding of and participation in various activities and sports. It is the intent of this Series to develop a more informed consumer and to stimulate widespread participation in a variety of activities and sports.

JACK H. WILMORE
Chairperson, Publications Committee
American College of Sports Medicine

# PREFACE

Bicycling is experiencing renewed popularity. Once again the bicycle has found its place in sport and culture. In its rebirth the bicycle has become more than a plaything of the aristocracy, a status symbol of the middle class, or an inexpensive tool for leisure pursuits. While maintaining its basic integrity as an efficient machine for human transport, it has been subject to existing technology. As the bicycle has been subjected to technological modification, riding technique and training too, have been the subject of scientific research.

The pioneer publication on the subject of cycling by Zuntz (1899) indicated an awareness of the complexity of cycling and the importance of physiological and biomechanical factors as they might affect the cyclist. This text represents a combined physiological and biomechanical approach to the sport of cycling. The text is intended to be of special interest to all enthusiastic cyclists. Portions of the book should meet the specific needs of cyclists and coaches in attempting to answer basic questions centering on the physiology and biomechanics of cycling.

This presentation represents an attempt to glean relevant facts from a variety of completed research and to apply them to the biomechanics and physiology of cycling. The primary intention has been to fill an apparent need for a publication that will bridge the chasm between the scientist and practitioner.

Within the recent past an amazing explosion of knowledge in exercise physiology and biomechanics of sports has occurred. Much of the

new knowledge, if not directly, certainly indirectly, is applicable
to cycling. Up until now, however, specific studies in the areas of the
exercise physiology and biomechanics of cycling have been very few in
number. This situation is now definitely improving but the implication
for the present monograph of the shortage of research material is that
the book will soon become outdated. This state of affairs can only be
good for the sport of cycling since, as more and more sport scientists
devote their energies toward cycling, a much better understanding of
the process will result. There will be several places where the reader
will notice an obvious void, where no specific guidance has been offered
on a particular topic. This is because we have tried to stay in the areas
where experimental evidence on which to base our statements is available. There are many publications on cycling where the opinions of
well-known authors are given on these topics and, until the experiments
are done, the reader will have to sift through the various shades of
opinion with their own critical eye. We have chosen to stay away from
these areas.

The aim of this volume is therefore twofold. First, the intention
is to provide a foundation of basic physiological and biomechanical
ideas that will give the cyclist a framework to interpret both personal
ideas and research studies that exist now and those reviewed in the
future. Second, a presentation of the relevant research findings to date
is given and the meaning of these findings for the cyclist is explained.
This will serve as an indication of the "state of the art" and form a
basis for the inclusion of new work in later editions. It will be apparent
to the cyclist that science has a long way to go to catch up with some
of the empirical data collected on a "trial and error" basis by the
cycling fraternity. However, if it is any consolation, science is moving
fast and the next few years will bring new information about physiological and biomechanical aspects of cycling.

The American College of Sports Medicine felt there was a need for a
volume on the physiology and biomechanics of cycling. It is our wish
that the knowledge presented will stimulate further investigation
leading to ways to extend the limits of human performance.

The authors are indebted to those researchers whose work is to be
discussed and referred to in this text. We wish to thank all who have
been associated with us in the various research endeavors on cycling.

IRVIN E. FARIA<br>
PETER R. CAVANAGH

# CONTENTS

# THE PHYSIOLOGY AND BIOMECHANICS OF CYCLING

# SECTION 1
# Science
# and the Cyclist

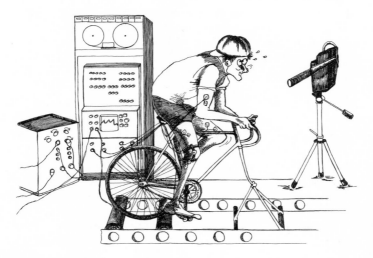

The physiology and biomechanics of sport have become an increasingly important topic for study and discussion. The push for scientific interest in a sport such as cycling is a result of the desire of coaches and athletes for better performance. The multiple phenomena involved in the physiology and biomechanics of cycling require close examination if optimum performance is to be achieved.

Physiology is the study of the function of the organism. Exercise or cycling physiology is concerned with the human functions under the stress of muscular activity as it relates to cycling. To this end it provides a basis for the study of training and adaptation to the sport of cycling.

The human organism is capable of performing extraordinary physical feats, even at the expense of temporarily losing internal equilibrium.

When insufficient amounts of oxygen are present, or when the oxygen-transport system is incapable of meeting the immediate needs, pre-programmed life-sustaining actions are initiated. In theory, the adaptation mechanism enables the working body to live temporarily beyond its capacity for oxygen transport to the active muscles and to compensate for so doing during recovery after exercise.

The need for studying the physiology of cycling can therefore be viewed as a need to provide an explanation of how the body responds and adapts to the work of cycling. Our first task is to examine its modus operandi and, once we have looked separately at the main functional components of the systems that affect adaptation to physical stress, we can put them together and see how the system works as a whole.

Although physiology may be a familiar term to many people, biomechanics may be something new. A satisfactory definition of biomechanics might be the following: "The use of objective techniques to analyze patterns of body movement, the timing of body movements, and the forces which create or result from movement."

To this definition we could add on other aspects of mechanics that are important in human movement. In the present context of cycling, these include such topics as friction, power output, strength of frame materials, properties of the transmission, and the properties of safety equipment, in addition to the mechanical aspects of the muscles and joints that are responsible for turning the pedals and steering the bicycle. It is clear that biomechanics is a very large "umbrella," and it is also true that cycling is more clearly a fusion of biology and mechanics than almost any other sport. The cyclist is completely dependent upon the mechanical aspects and functioning of the machine and, as we will see in later sections on energy supply, there is a finite limit to the steady-state power that can be delivered by human metabolism. The cyclist is faced with a number of major forms of resistance that consume this valuable metabolic power output; the way in which power is dissipated will influence who will win the race or who will be able to complete a tour with least fatigue. An understanding of certain mechanical phenomena and the motivation to put this insight to work while out riding the bicycle can allow each individual to make optimum use of their own physiological attributes and conditioning level.

The necessity for a look at the biomechanics of cycling can therefore be stated as a need to provide a description of how the body applies power to the bicycle, and how the external forces combine to oppose the cyclist. We have probably all had the experience of being faced with the repair of an appliance that we know absolutely nothing about. The first stage is usually to find out how it functions and, once that is grasped, repair and subsequent operation of the device are simplified. The same principles apply to cycling; if we understand—in a general way—how our musculoskeletal system is functioning and what the mechanics of the rider-environment interface are, then we are more likely to be better cyclists—safer and more efficient.

We start in the remainder of this section with a description of some of the techniques of study that have been used to understand the physiology and biomechanics of cycling. If you are mainly interested in the results and not' in how they were obtained, see Section 2.

Subsequent sections will aim to achieve four objectives: (1) to describe the human engine in terms of a biological and mechanical machine for producing power; (2) to provide insight into the resistances in cycling that the human power output is directed against; (3) to present in a readable manner the results of research studies that have relevance to efficient cycling; and (4) to discuss some considerations regarding injury and outline some necessary precautions in order to safely enjoy the sport of cycling.

## THE TECHNIQUES OF STUDY

The tools of the trade for biomechanists are many and varied. Here we will introduce you to the most important ones so that they will already be familiar to you when they appear subsequently sections.

**THE BICYCLE ERGOMETER, ROLLERS, AND THE TREAD-MILL.** Studying the cyclist out on the road is not easy, although many experimenters have been brave enough to try. Most of us have taken the easy way out and have brought the cyclist into the laboratory to ride either a bicycle ergometer or a standard bicycle mounted on rollers or on the treadmill. The ergometer has been used most widely in physiological tests. It generally has a standard fixed wheel transmission that drives a large flywheel. In a crude way, the flywheel simulates the momentum that the cyclist would have out on the road. Since a friction brake is applied to the flywheel, pedalling can be made more difficult by calibrated and reproducable amounts. The device has no wheels and its handlebars, saddle, and pedals are often rather differently positioned than on a normal bicycle. For this reason cyclists frequently say that they feel uncomfortable on the ergometer and, more importantly, that they do things differently when riding it. Therefore, it is preferable to

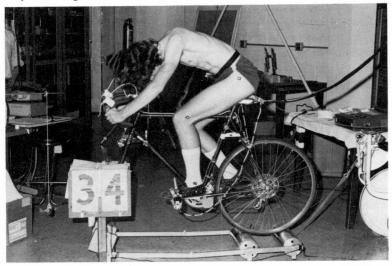

**FIGURE 1.1.** Typical experimental setup for a biomechanical study of cycling where the front forks of a racing bicycle are supported on a frame and the rear wheel rests on friction braked rollers.

study cyclists riding their own bicycles. Rollers are effective for this purpose, as shown in Figure 1.1.

The rear wheel of the bicycle sits between two rollers of about five inches in diameter and, as the cyclist pedals, a belt drive causes a single roller under the front wheel to rotate, giving a similar gyroscopic effect to that which occurs out on the road. There is quite a skill factor to riding rollers, and naive subjects often feel more at home if the bicycle is held upright by a helper or better still by a frame supporting the front wheel. Providing a standard work load with rollers is a little more difficult than on an ergometer. First, factors such as tire pressures will make a difference, and second, most rollers have low friction bearings and no means of applying resistance. However, a friction brake can be improvised. The final alternative for eliminating forward motion is to put the rider on a treadmill. At first this feels like riding across a frozen lake without brakes but, with practice and acute concentration, the skill can be mastered.

Now that we have prevented the cyclist from pedaling into the distance, we are ready to apply further techniques to study the mechanics of cycling.

**HIGH-SPEED CINEMATOGRAPHY.** It may come as a surprise that the movie camera can be a scientific measuring instrument but it certainly can! Although the human eye is perhaps our most valuable sense organ, it is badly equipped for discerning the fine characteristics of fast movement. Simple observation by eye has in the past led to some very erroneous ideas about foot action in cycling as we will see in a later section on ankling. With a suitable cine camera, images that are typically only several thousandths of a second apart can be obtained; these images can be replayed one frame at a time, as if we had hundreds of still photographs. Alternatively, a continuous, slow-motion replay can be achieved. In the present context, certain anatomical landmarks on the subject are usually marked to allow more precise measurement to be made, and these lead to rather complete and accurate information about the motion of the joints of the body. When plotted out in graphical form, the results allow easy interpretation and understanding of patterns of joint and body segment motion.

**FORCE AND TORQUE MEASUREMENT.** When observing the motion of the limbs, even high-speed cinematography can only go so far toward explaining what the body is doing during cycling. In some ways, measuring the motion of the limb segments is like seeing smoke and trying to guess what is burning; you can get some indication, but the result will almost always be inconclusive. A much more definitive and useful method is to actually measure the external force that muscular action is creating. The techniques for doing this are very sophisticated electrical measurements that take advantage of the fact that most structures are not completely rigid and therefore deform under the action of a force. If the deformation can be measured, the magnitude of the force can be implied. Devices called "strain gauges" are glued firmly to structures such as the crank or specially designed pedals (see Section 7). As these structures deform, (even only a few thousandths of an inch), the gauges also deform and the measuring equipment gives a continuous output of force or torque depending upon the situation. It becomes possible, as we will see later, to determine exactly how a cyclist is applying force at a particular point in the cycle, and this can be very useful as far as the determination of efficient pedalling is concerned.

**ELECTROMYOGRAPHY.** Most people are fairly familiar with the electrocardiograph, a device used by the cardiologist to help evaluate the condition of the heart. The signals that are detected with this equipment result from electrical activity in the heart, which is really just a muscular bag. In much the same way, the muscles that are attached to the skeleton also have electrical activity associated with their action. With the right equipment these electrical signals can be detected despite the fact that they are only a few thousandths of a volt in size.

This technique, electromyography, is not usually used to diagnose the quality of the muscle (although it can be used for this purpose in cases of muscle disease). It is generally used to give some indication of which muscle groups are active during a given part of the pedalling cycle. This technique does not have a great practical importance, but it is instrumental in gaining a more complete insight into the mechanism of pedalling.

**WIND TUNNELS.** In Section 6 we will confirm that on level ground the resistance offered by the air—called drag— is the principal enemy of the cyclist. Bringing the cyclist into the laboratory and using one of the methods described earlier to make the bicycle stationary is, of course, an effective way of eliminating drag. Since an intimate knowledge of the major enemy is the best ammunition in any conflict, techniques must be devised to learn more about the effects of drag. Some ingenious experiments have been done outdoors using other cyclists as windshields, or getting riders to freewheel down hills in different riding postures. (These are experiments that the interested reader might want to replicate with a stopwatch.)

By far the most controlled method of studying the effects of drag has been stolen from aeronautical engineering. It can be shown theoretically that the effects on an object moving in a fluid (such as air) are identical if the object is held stationary and the fluid is moved past at the speed with which the object was originally travelling. The idea then is to mount a bike and rider inside a large tunnel and blow air toward them at speeds comparable to a range of riding speeds. If the bike is restrained from moving backward under the force of the wind by a force-measuring device, an indication of the effect of different riding postures upon drag can be obtained. We will see later that some surprising findings have resulted from experiments of this kind.

**USE OF EXPERIMENTAL DISTURBANCES.** To study how a cyclist reacts to a sudden gust of wind would take a rather long time if the experimenter had to wait for exactly the right wind—from the right direction and of the right magnitude. Some elegant experiments have been conducted in which small rockets were attached to the bicycle frame. At the whim of the experimenter, these rockets could be fired and the response of the unsuspecting human guinea pig to a calibrated disturbance could be studied. All this may sound a little exotic and far removed from you riding your bike to the office each day. However, such studies have proved useful in specifying more about the interaction of the rider and the machine.

**MATHEMATICAL MODELLING.** More than we might realize, this nice piece of jargon—the mathematical model—already plays an important part in our day-to-day lives. Particularly in the field of economics and fiscal policies, decisions are often made not on the basis of what actually happens, but as a result of what a collection of complex mathematical equations predict will happen in the future.

A mathematical model can be thought of as a black box (usually in the form of a computer program), which is fed a certain amount of initial data describing a system under scrutiny. After some digestion, this black box divulges a response that should be quite close to what actually happens to the system in real life. You might reasonably ask: Why bother with the model? Well, it is useful because the effect of many different initial conditions can be studied without the need to wait for the exact situation to occur in real life. A simple mathematical model might give us a prediction, for instance, of how long it would take you to drop with exhaustion while trying to ride up a 15 percent grade. You would surely appreciate being spared the task of actually having to attempt to ride!

We will briefly meet the predictions of some mathematical models of cycling later. At present, you might feel comforted to know that they usually don't work 100 percent perfectly. The human subject generally manages to confound the most exact mathematical description!

**LINKING BIOMECHANICS AND PHYSIOLOGY.** Perhaps the most potent form of biomechanical experiment is one that has been attempted only rarely up until now. It involves making some change to the mechanics of the riding situation, such as changing the pedalling action or the seat height, and measuring what the change does to the metabolism of the cyclist. This must be the ultimate laboratory test concerning our speculation about what is best and what is most efficient. Any proposed modification that results, for example, in increased oxygen consumption under similar riding conditions, must be discounted, and one that causes decreased consumption should be encouraged. Later we will describe the results of a few of these studies but generally scientists have ignored this fruitful line of approach.

The preceding material will have acquainted you with biomechanics and physiology. In subsequent sections, we will describe the results of studies on cyclists and their bicycles that used the techniques described here. The brief descriptions included here will make the results more understandable and more meaningful.

## SOME BACKGROUND READING IN BIOMECHANICS AND EXERCISE PHYSIOLOGY

We hope that the reader will be stimulated to draw on other sources as a result of the brief exposure that is given here. For those with more that just a passing interest in the scientific aspects of cycling, we recommend the book, *Bicycling Science—Ergonomics and Mechanics,* by Whitt and Wilson (1974). Another facinating book, perhaps the largest treatise on the mechanical aspects of cycling ever written, is *Bicycles and Tricycles* by A. Sharpe, which was published in 1894 and still contains many items of more than just historical interest. For the reader who feels the need for a more general grounding in biomechanics as it applies to sport, *The Biomechanics of Sports Techniques* by James Hay (1973) provides some very readable accounts of various concepts but does not deal with any problems related to cycling. *The Biology of Physical Activity* by Edington and Edgerton (1976) will benefit the reader who wishes more backgound knowledge in exercise physiology. Be aware of the publications, *Bike World* and *Bicycling,* both of which from time to time have very relevant articles on biomechanical, medical, and physiological aspects of cycling. Finally, a good primer for everything from components to cycling folklore is *Delong's Guide to Bicycles and Bicycling,* which distills the experience of a veteran enthusiast into a readable form.

## BIBLIOGRAPHY

*Bicycling.* Published monthly by Capital Management Publications, 119 Paul Drive, P. O. Box 3330, San Rafael, Calif. 94902.

*Bike World.* Published monthly by World Publications, Box 366, Mountain View, Calif. 94040.

DeLong, Fred. *DeLong's Guide to Bicycles and Bicycling.* Chilton Book Co., Radnor, Pa. 1974.

Edington, D. W., and V. R. Edgerton. *The Biology of Physical Acticity.* Houghton Mifflin Co., Boston. 1976.

Hay, James G. *The Biomechanics of Sports Techniques.* Prentice Hall, Englewood Cliffs, N. J. 1973.

Sharpe, A. *Bicycles and Tricycles.* Longmans, Green and Co., London. 1894.

Whitt, F. R., and D. G. Wilson. *Bicycling Science: Ergonomics and Mechanics.* M. I. T. Press, Cambridge, Mass. 1974.

# SECTION 2
# Supply and Demand

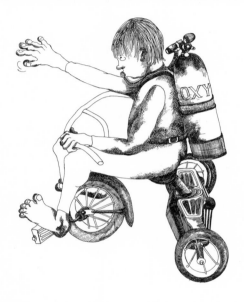

This section will serve to provide essential background information. Basic concepts, principles, and functions presented here will be alluded to later. We will concentrate on energy, its source, production, and use. To both the cyclist and cycling coach, a basic knowledge of the bioenergetics of cycling is extremely important if sound training practices and competitive riding plans are to be developed. For a better understanding and appreciation of the events that take place within the cycling body, we explore the working muscle, its energy supply and demand.

In the world we live, energy is transformed from one type to another. Energy is defined as the capacity to do work. Work is often defined as the product of a given force acting through a given distance. There are, however, different kinds of work as there are different kinds of energy. Mechanically, work is the product of force and displacement; however, physiologically, living cells use chemical energy to perform chemical work or what might be considered internal work. The primary energy source for life and movement is the sun (See Figure 2.1). The small amount of light energy reaching the earth is

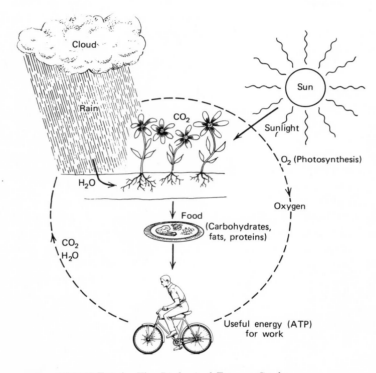

**FIGURE 2.1.** The Biological Energy Cycle.

converted by green plants into chemical energy in the form of sugars, which are carbohydrates. The energy conversion process, known as photosynthesis, not only produces essential carbohydrates as an energy source but also produces oxygen. Human beings cannot produce chemical energy in the form of carbohydrates or sugars; therefore, they and other animals are dependent on eating plants that produce sugars or on eating other animals who have eaten plants. The energy trapped in the sugars by photosynthesis is released in the muscle cell by a series of chemical reactions or oxidations. Finally, the energy initially derived from the sun is used by the animal to perform chemical work.

Oxidation is the addition of oxygen to a compound or element, the removal of electrons from an atom, or the removal of hydrogen from a compound. Each of these three processes take place within the muscle cell. Basically, the process involves the breaking of high-energy chemical bonds and the removal of hydrogen atoms, which combine with oxygen to form water and energy for muscle contraction. In the process, carbon dioxide is formed and released along with heat.

When food materials are eaten, digested, absorbed, and delivered by the blood to the muscle cell, certain molecular particles enter the cell. Within the cell wall and cell proper a complex chain of biochemical reactions take place that produce energy. By way of several biochemical pathways the muscle cell gains energy. These include the aerobic and mitrochondrial electron pathway, and the anaerobic (lactic-acid producing) pathway.

Each of us is composed of a hundred trillion cells or more. With each movement the body requires the collaboration of thousands of nerve and muscle cells. The muscle cell in particular shows a remarkable ability for obtaining and using energy. Exploring the interior structure and function of the muscle cell is an exciting beginning to the appreciation, knowledge, and understanding of the cycling body.

For a few moments allow us to draw a concept from Isaac Asimov, author of *Fantastic Voyage* and, through the process of miniaturization, enter into the microuniverse of a single muscle cell. As we approach a billionth of our normal size, we are injected into the femoral artery of the right leg. Upon entering the blood stream, we are swept away like a fallen log in a rushing river during a torrential rainstorm. Quickly we are carried in the blood plasma toward the large thigh muscle, the vastus medialis.

Within a few minutes our movement velocity lessens, and up ahead we can see what appears to be a structure resembling a fish net. As the blood vessel narrows, it is clear now that we are entering a capillary bed that lies close to the muscle fibers. Now and then we are nudged by red blood cells until finally being lodged between two red cells as we pass into a capillary. Some dizziness is experienced that is due to the mixing motion of the plasma flow. This action appears to speed up the equilibration of gases, oxygen, and carbon dioxide between the blood and muscle tissue. Inching our way through the capillary, we find ourselves about to come to a stop; then suddenly we pass through the porous wall of the capillary. Passing through the wall, we can feel the movement of carbon dioxide molecules against us while oxygen molecules help push us across the capillary membrane.

In a millisecond we enter into the muscle cell. The quickness of our entry was indeed enhanced by the surface to an interplumbinglike system called the T system. Inside the cell and bathed in a sea of fluid called cytoplasm are several large and complex structures or molecules. To gain a better perspective of these special organs or organelles, we climb to the top of the cell's heredity-bearing core, the nucleus. From our new vantage point we can observe certain organelles performing their life-sustaining tasks. However, our first observation is that within the cytoplasm itself, enzymes are busy at work producing a chemical called ATP, or adenosine triphosphate. All energy is produced by means of enzymes. These enzymes have a special function in promoting biological reactions. A general trait of a living system is the ability to rapidly oxidize glucose at moderate temperatures. Enzymes function to increase the rate of chemical reactions. The working muscle cell needs more than two million molecules of ATP a second to drive its biochemical processes. The production of ATP is essentially controlled by enzyme activity. The processes are greatly enhanced by another plumbing system, the scarcoplasmic reticulum. This network is seen to reside in the narrow spaces between the myofibrils, which are the contractual units of muscle action. In this vast plumbing system, we can see substances required for metabolism moving through it.

Floating in the cytoplasm are bean-shaped organelles whose primary function is observed to be that of converting sugar and fat derivatives into energy for the cell's use. These dynamos or powerhouses are the mitochondria. Electrons and hydrogen ions from the broken-down compounds are seen to pass along an enzyme assembly line. As they pass along, their energy is packaged into energy-rich bundles of ATP. This ATP will later be used to provide energy for muscle contraction. In the process of energy production it is quite apparent that the mitochondria are taking up oxygen. As an oxygen using structure, mitochrondria are responsible for aerobic muscular work.

During our short journey into the muscle cell a most significant observation has been made. The muscle cell is capable of energy transformation, which may be accomplished with or without the use of oxygen.

Cycling may be performed aerobically or anaerobically. The concept of aerobic work implies that the rate of oxygen uptake is adequate to meet the oxygen needs of the working body cells as they use substrates of carbohydrates and fats for energy. Lower-intensity, long-duration cycling at a steady state of energy utilization is an example of aerobic work. When the work intensity is such that an adequate supply of oxygen is not available to support the energy demand, the effort is anaerobic. During anaerobic work limited quantities of stored energy are drawn upon. A cyclist can perform at top speed for not more than 10 to 30 seconds anaerobically. Consequently, anaerobic performance is at a high intensity but short duration.

Regardless of the energy producing pathway utilized, aerobic or anaerobic, energy in the form of adenosine triphosphate (ATP) is generated. Adenosine phosphates are involved in the capture of energy in the form of high-energy phosphate bonds. When food materials are oxidized, chemical bonds are broken, thereby removing hydrogen atoms and releasing carbon dioxide. The fracturing of the chemical bonds results in the release of energy that went into their formation as well as the loss of some energy as heat. Released energy that went into bond formation is captured to be either immediately used or stored by the cell. The intracellular energy-capturing molecule is ATP. In turn, ATP releases its energy when it is enzymatically broken down to its previous structure (ADP and Pi).

The energy for cycling is provided by means of one of three chemical or metabolic systems: (1) the ATP-CP system, (2) the lactic-acid system, and (3) the oxygen system. Each system serves in a specific manner to provide energy for muscle contraction (Figure 2.2). Each in its own way uniquely contributes to the energy base of the muscle cell, and each holds a significance for the cyclist.

The ATP-CP system is cetilized for power starts of sprints and breakaways that require only a few seconds to complete. During the short explosive period of cycling, about 8 to 10 seconds, the muscle depends upon ATP generation through a rapid combustion or one-enzyme reaction. Enzymes exist in both the cytoplasm and the mitochondria of the muscle cell. They start chemical reactions without un-

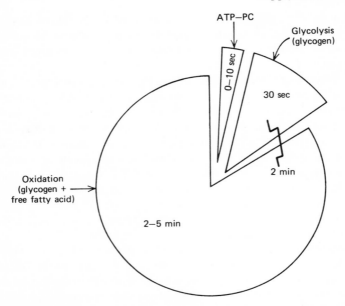

**FIGURE 2.2.** Time-dependent sequence of the activation of energy sources within an active muscle.

dergoing any self-modification. All enzymes are proteins, and several have an additional, nonprotein portion called a coenzyme. Which compound an enzyme will influence is dictated by its protein portion. The active portion of the starter or catalyst is the coenzyme that is essential in carrying out a reaction. Vitamins, trace elements, and pigments have been identified as coenzymes. The B vitamins, for example, are essential coenzymes for carbohydrate metabolism. A rise in muscle cell temperature increases enzyme activity. Thus, warm-up prior to intense cycling is beneficial, since it is conducive to more rapid adaptation to the oncoming work and theoretically allows for more rapid production of energy (ATP). Within the muscle cell an enzyme, creatine phosphokinase, stimulates the chemical action to produce energy (ATP) from creatine phosphate (CP). This energy producing reaction is accomplished by the linking of adenosine diphosphate (ADP) with a third phosphate (Pi) to form adenosine triphosphate (ATP). This enzymatic action will continue until the muscle has exhausted itself of the creatine phosphate supply. Until then, cellular ATP is transported throughout the muscle cell to meet the energy needs of the cell. The maximum amount of energy that may be derived from depletion of the alactic sources has been estimated to be approximately 100 calories per kilogram of body weight. This estimate is for very heavy cycling leading to exhaustion in a few minutes.

The extremely rapid synthesis of ATP is enhanced by another enzyme, adenylate kinase. This enzyme indirectly stimulates the initiation of a reaction that leads to the mobilization of short-term energy. Without such an energy producing system, high-speed cycling would be impossible because of the delay in the transporting of oxygen to the muscle when work is begun.

Like the other systems, this short-term energy producing system is only as effective as the weakest part of the system. That is, the speed of the chain of chemical processes is governed by the speed of the slower, single reaction in the series.

Because this ATP-CP system is time-dependent, identified as 0 to 10 seconds, a training protocol should be structured within the time zone to sufficiently overload the system. Research suggests that with proper training, the enzymatic reactions may be enhanced.

The lactic-acid system or anaerobic pathway serves as an energy source for cycling periods of approximately 30 seconds to 2 minutes. The mechanism involved is glycolysis, which means the "dissolving of sugar." Energy production through this system involves the use of glucose or glycogen for the manufacture of ATP. Glucose is the major sugar molecule making up starches and glycogens. During intense cycling, stored intramuscular glycogen is broken down non-oxidatively to form ATP and lactic acid. In the absence of oxygen, glucose is only partially broken down by means of a series of enzymes that direct a succession of structure changes of the glucose molecule to lactic acid, a by-product of glycolysis. Lactic acid accumulates when not enough oxygen can be supplied to serve the metabolic needs of the working muscles. When there is a lack of oxygen, the chemical reactions are not completed; thus electrons from the electron-transport system accumulate. This electron accumulation increases as the body depends more and more on glycolysis for energy. The result is that the normal products of glycolysis are unable to enter the Krebs cycle, a series of chemical reactions; therefore, lactate is the end product. With high-intensity cycling the production of lactic acid soon exceeds the body's capacity to break it down. The accumulation of lactate modifies the cell environment to the point where the acid state will not allow other molecules to function. Depletion of muscle glycogen plus the lactic acid accumulation results in the condition commonly known as fatigue.

As is true for all energy producing systems, the speed of a single biochemical reaction of glycolysis is governed by both the amount of fuel available, in this case glucose and glycogen, and the effectiveness of the catalyst or enzyme system. The significance of this chemical law for the cyclist is that training must involve the stressing of all the enzyme and fuel systems. In response to stress produced from overloading the system, the fuel system will become programmed to work at an increased rate.

It is interesting to note that a glucose molecule undergoing glycolysis will net two ATP molecules. Although this is only 5 percent of the total yield derived when the same amount of glucose is completely broken down to carbon dioxide ($CO_2$) and water ($H_2O$) in the presence of oxygen, it allows the cyclist to perform at extremely high intensity for about two minutes. At the conclusion of the intense work, the lactate molecules can either be utilized by the muscle to form $CO_2$ and $H_2O$ or be transported to the liver. In the liver, two lactate molecules can be converted to a glucose molecule. The glucose is then either stored as glycogen in the liver or released into the blood stream and transported to the muscle for its utilization.

The oxygen system or aerobic pathway (Krebs cycle plus the electron-transport chain) is employed for the long-term source of energy. This is a metabolic process whereby oxygen is used to generate a total of 38 molecules of ATP through the complete breakdown of a glucose molecule. The system generates ATP by coupling the utilization of oxygen, needed to power the electron transport system, with the oxidation of hydrogen carriers in the electron-transport sytsem. The system is dependent upon the cardiorespiratory system to furnish it with oxygen by means of hemoglobin in the blood. If sufficient oxygen is supplied to meet the metabolic demands, lactic acid does not accumulate.

In order to attempt to meet oxygen demands, the heart rate and respiration volume increase. The respiratory system serves two important functions during energy production. First, it eliminates from the body $CO_2$ produced in the Krebs cycle. Second, it extracts oxygen from the air. The cardiovascular system, however, is not the main limiting factor for aerobic cycling work. Instead, cellular oxygen utilization is probably the main limiting factor for aerobic power.

A derivative of acetic acid or vinegar called acetyle-SCoA is the fuel that produces ATP by means of the Krebs cycle. Acetyl-SCoA is generated from the breakdown of carbohydrates and fats. Also essential for the functioning of this aerobic system is a continuing supply of hydrogen carriers. These carriers arise from fatty acid oxidation and the oxidation of acetyl-SCoA in the Krebs cycle.

When the body's glycogen supply is depleted at the end of about a 200-kilometer, hard ride, the body turns to fats in the form of free fatty acids (FFA) as a fuel. Fats are broken down to acetyl-SCoA by a process called oxidation and scission. The final end products of this process—ATP, water, and heat—are the result of the action of a series of enzymes and cytochromes (electron-transport chain) that use the available oxygen.

The oxidation and scission process of the Krebs cycle and electron-transport system is rather slow, and therefore unable to provide energy for high-intensity cycling. Through training, however, it is possible to condition and program the system to break down and use fat as a major source of fuel at high rates of speed. Long-term, steady-state riding will enhance the potential of fat as a fuel.

In summary, the extent to which the various energy source systems are utilized depends on the intensity and duration of cycling. There exists a well-ordered relationship between energy supply and demand. Supramaximal, short-term cycling is dependent on the alactic system; high-intensity, short period work calls upon the anaerobic system, and prolonged cycling draws on the aerobic system. No one energy-producing-source system exists independently but each interlocks with the other proving an ongoing energy source to meet the generated demands (See Figure 2.3).

## BIBLIOGRAPHY

Asimov, I. *Fantastic Voyage.* Gorgi Books, London. 1966.

Asimov, I. *Life and Energy.* Bantam Books, New York. 1965.

Åstrand, P. O., and K. Rodahl. *Textbook of work Physiology.*
    (McGraw-Hill, New York. 1970.

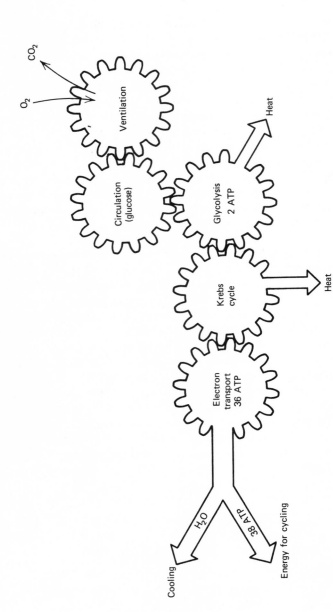

**FIGURE 2.3.** General view of the major biochemical pathways; glycolysis, Krebs cycle, and electron transport system.

*Goldsby, R. A. Cells and Energy.* The MacMillan Company, New York. 1969.

Keul, J. (editor). *Limiting Factors of Physical Performance.* George Thieme Publishers, Stuttgart. 1973.

Lehninger, A. L. *Bioenergetics. W. A. Benjamin, New York. 1965.*

Mathews, D. K., and E. L. Fox. *The Physiological Basis of Physical Education and Athletics.* W. B. Saunders Company, Philadelphia 1971.

Racker, E. *Mechanisms in Bioenergetics.* Academic Press, New York 1965.

# SECTION 3
# What are My Muscles Doing?

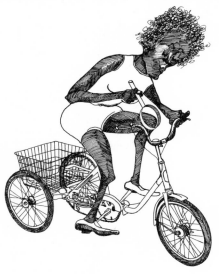

This section describes how your muscles produce force; it is organized so that you can make your own decision about how deeply you want to delve into the mechanism of muscle action. In much the same way as an automobile manufacturer provides a workshop manual for the mechanic and an owner's manual for the driver of a car, Part 1 explains in some detail what the various parts look like, what modifies their performance, and what their theory of operation is; Part 1 then is the workshop manual and you should read it only if you want to get some inside knowledge on why muscles work the way they do. The effort will be well worth it because, without this knowledge, it is difficult to understand what gearing is all about or why seat height

23

makes a difference. If you are looking for an outline of how the finished product works and where to find the major parts, then you
should flip through the first part of this section and begin reading
"Part 2-The Muscle Owner's Manual."

# PART I—THE
# WORKSHOP MANUAL
# FOR MUSCLE

When we see a cyclist in smooth, powerful motion during a race or
time trial, it is hard to imagine that the basic events causing the motion
of his or her limbs are happening at a level some 1000 times smaller
than the unaided eye can see. Figure 3.1 shows various parts of this
force generating mechanism, starting from surface features and pro-
gressing with successive increases in magnification until the fundamental unit of force production is schematically shown. Figure 3.1$a$ is a
photograph of the prominent calf muscle called the gastrocnemius
("belly of the leg") taken while the cyclist was midway through the
power stroke with this leg. From the photograph, it is apparent (1)
that the fleshy part of the muscle ends about one-third of the way
down between knee and ankle and (2) that there seem to be two
distinct parts to the muscle. If the skin, subcutaneous fascia, and fat
were removed from this leg, the appearance would be similar to that
shown in Figure 3.1$b$. The basic gross structure of this muscle is fairly
typical of skeletal muscle in the body; the muscular tissue is sand-
wiched between a tendon at either end, and it is the tendon that has a
secure attachment to parts of the skeleton. Through evolution of the
species and growth and development of the individual, the places
where many important tendons insert into bone have raised prominen-
cies on the bony structures that we call tubercles, tuberosities, and
other names depending upon their size and location.

The long tendon that runs from the termination of the fleshy part
of the gastrocnemius to the calcaneus or heel bone is known as the
Achilles tendon and is amongst the strongest of tendons in the body.
At the upper end of the muscle, the tendons are quite different in
character; the muscle divides into two parts, confirming the impression
derived from the surface anatomy, and only a short length of tendon
follows the termination of the fleshy part of the muscle. However,

some slips of tendon do begin lower down toward the belly of the muscle. This dissection of the leg would also have revealed other important structures; in particular, arteries, veins, and nerves would be visible travelling both beneath the muscle and over its exposed surface.

Taking a small slice from the belly of the muscle would result in the specimen shown in Figure 3.1c, where a further level of organization is apparent. It is here that we meet the single muscle cell called the muscle fiber, which is grouped together with many other similar fibers into the bundles or fasciculi seen in the diagram. With patience and keen eyesight, one of these bundles could be teased apart to leave a single muscle fiber which, despite being several inches long, is only about two hundredths of an inch thick. It is at this stage that the eye needs assistance; a small sample, taken from one of the fasciculi, might result in parts of three single muscle fibers shown schematically in Figure 3.1d as they would appear under a light microscope. At this stage some histochemical procedures would identify whether the muscle fibers were fast-or slow-twitch fibers, with the consequences for sprint or endurance performance that are mentioned in Section 8.

Although it is drawn in this diagram, the most important structure to the survival and function of the muscle cell would not be visible under the light microscope. This is the cell membrane or sarcolemma, which both encloses the cell like an envelope and possesses an intricate network of communicating passages called the sarcoplasmic reticulum, which permeate throughout the inner part of the fiber. As well as regulating the metabolism of the cell, which is the function of all cell membranes, the sarcolemma possesses the vital property of being electrically excitable. Injury, the action of certain chemical substances, or electrical stimulation will cause a brief and reversible change in electrical potential to spread throughout the sarcolemma and sarcoplasmic reticulum. During activity of the kind shown in Figure 3.1a, electrical impulses are arriving through the nerve fibers at rates of up to 50 impulses per second, and each impulse is the trigger for a fascinating chain of events that has needed clever deduction and the electron microscope to unravel. As we will see later, the electrical impulse that precedes every period of force production and the resulting electrical change in the sarcolemma are relatively simple to detect from a living person by placing electrodes over or inside a muscle such as the gastrocnemius. This technique, called electromyography

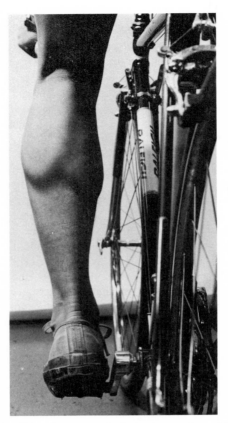

**FIGURE 3.1.a** The elements of skeletal muscle, with increasing magnification as the parts being examined get smaller.

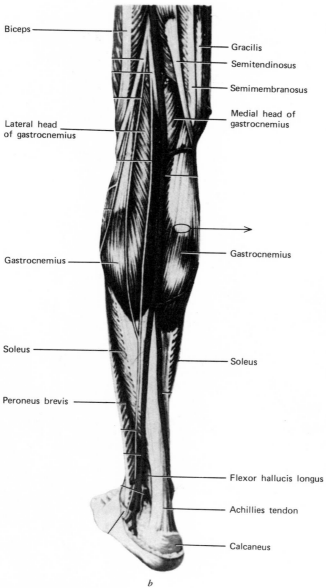

Biceps

Gracilis
Semitendinosus
Semimembranosus

Lateral head
of gastrocnemius

Medial head of
gastrocnemius

Gastrocnemius

Gastrocnemius

Soleus

Soleus

Peroneus brevis

Flexor hallucis longus

Achillies tendon

Calcaneus

*b*

**FIGURE 3.1.b (Continued)**

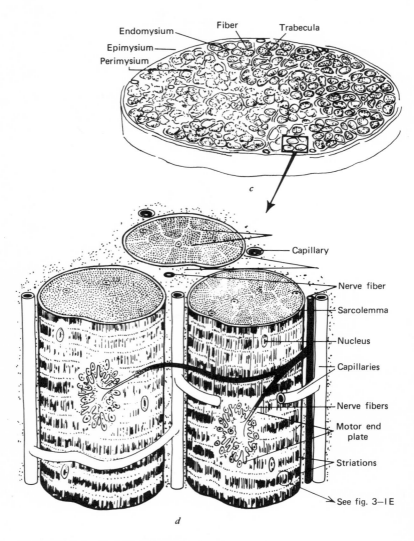

FIGURE 3.1.c & d (Continued)

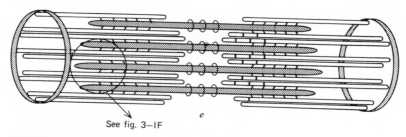

See fig. 3-1F

**FIGURE 3.1.e (Continued)**

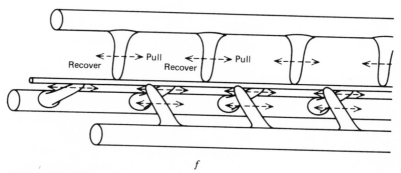

Recover ← - - → Pull ← - - → Pull Recover ← - - → ← - - → ← - - →

*f*

**FIGURE 3.1.f (Continued)**

(see Section 1), can be used to give an indication of which muscle groups are active during cycling or other movements.

Also shown in Figure 3.1d are small blood vessels, the capillaries, in which certain metabolic energy sources and waste products flow together with blood at rest or during a weak contraction. There would be a considerably greater number of these surrounding the slow-twitch than the fast-twitch fibers. However, when the muscle is producing more than a modest amount of force, the capillaries are literally squashed by adjacent muscle fibers that increase their diameter as they are activated. This aids the return of blood to the heart by acting as a simple pump but, in prolonged muscular action, it also results in fatigue, since no blood flows through the active tissue. The electromyographic evidence indicates, as we will see, that the activity of the major lower-limb muscles in cycling can be characterized by short phases of activity followed by a period of rest. This pattern of activity results in temporary occlusion of blood flow followed by a restoration of normal flow.

An important feature that would be recognized through the light microscope is the banding or striation that is seen across the length of the fiber (Figure 3.1d). The cross section reveals a further suborganization of small structures called myofibrils, and it is within these structures that the important events of muscular activity occur. The structure of one element of a single myofibril is shown schematically in Figure 3.1e. The striations are seen to be the result of two kinds of filaments which, when they overlap, produce a dark band. It is clear from the figure that all the myofibrils have their overlapping regions approximately in line to give the whole fiber a striped appearance. One complete set of these repeating patterns at the single fiber level is called a sarcomere, and the length of a typical sarcomere is approximately one thousandth of an inch (2.5 microns). If we go one further step down in size, we have finally arrived at the location of force production.

The two different sized sets of rods shown in Figure 3.1e should really be shown as chains of protein molecules; the thin filaments composed mainly of a protein called actin and the thick filaments composed of myosin. Actin has a structure like two lengths of beads wound around each other, while myosin has a more complex, helical structure. The arrival of the change in electrical potential at the sarcolemma cause the two different proteins to begin a complex interaction that is shown schematically in Figure 3.1f.

Projections from the thick filaments attach to specific sites on the actin chain for a very brief period of time. During this period of attachment it is believed that the actin chain is drawn past the myosin chain, and the whole cycle repeats when the projection or cross bridge reattaches to a site further along the actin chain. All of the bridges shown in the figure would not be active together, and the random making and breaking of the connections ensures that a steady tension can be exerted at the ends of the sarcomere. One critical point is that there is a strict directionality to the motion of the cross bridges. Those in the upper part of the sarcomere can only pull the actin filaments downward and those in the lower portion can only attempt to pull the actin filaments upward. If this was not the case, a muscle would be able to push as well as pull.

This is an appropriate point to mention that the term muscular contraction is somewhat of a misnomer. Although the muscle is receiving electrical impulses and the bridges are being made between the two kinds of protein filaments, the effect will be to try and bring the ends of the sarcomere closer together. If the attempt is successful, then shortening or contraction does occur and we say that the muscle is acting *concentrically*. However, the ends of the sarcomere may be firmly fixed, resulting in the development of a static force between the points of attachment—an *isometric* force (literally the same length). Finally, an external force may be acting to lengthen the sarcomere and, despite a maximal effort, the cross bridges are not able to produce enough force to halt the lengthening; this would be an example of *eccentric* action. Clearly, to call all three of these conditions contraction will result in an erroneous statement in two out of three cases.

## THE EFFECT OF LENGTH ON MUSCLE FORCE

The amount of tension that a muscle produces is directly proportional to the number of active cross bridges. When the unit shown in Figure 3.1e is drawn out so that there is very little overlap, only a few binding sites are available and little tension can be developed. At the other extreme, two factors affect the development of tension when the sarcomere length is small. First, since there are no cross bridges in the middle of the myosin filament, the degree of overlap shown in Figure 3.1e represents the optimum condition where most force can be developed. Second, as the ends of the sarcomere get even closer together than shown, there comes a point where the thick filaments physically butt up against the end of the sarcomere, and this reduces

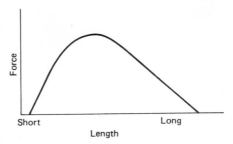

**FIGURE 3.2a.** Changes in force output as the length of an individual sarcomere is altered.

force output almost to zero.

The situation at the sarcomere is therefore like the inverted "U" shown in Figure 3.2a. There is a length at which maximum tension can be developed, and both above and below this length tension falls off. Now it is clear from Figure 3.1 that a complete, anatomical muscle like the gastrocnemius consists of thousands of fibers, each composed of thousands of myofibrils, and that each myofibril consists of thousands of units like that in Figure 3.1e, joined end to end or in series. A typical muscle is capable of shortening about two or three inches and, since each sarcomere can only shorten about half of its own resting length (about 1.25 microns or 0.0005 inches), there must be at least 5000 sarcomeres in the muscle fibers of a large muscle.

When this whole muscle is at a short length, the argument outlined above for the sarcomere is directly applicable. A short muscle is not in a very favorable position to develop tension. At the longer lengths, the sarcomere argument does not hold because the tendons together with some of the structures shown in Figure 3.1e, called the epimysium, perimysium, and endomysium, affect the total tension that is developed. These structures are connective tissue that enclose the complete muscle, the fasciculi, and the single fibers, as well as being interconnected with each other. At each end of the muscle these connective tissue structures merge with the tendon as does the membrane of the individual fibers. When the muscle is stretched, the effect of the connective tissue is similar to that of a strong spring. Regardless of what the protein machinery is doing, there is energy stored in the "spring" that exerts a strong force, attempting to shorten the muscle. This means that at longer lengths, the maximum tension that a muscle can exert actually increases despite the fact that the contractile machinery is placed in a disadvantageous position for force development. Therefore, if we were able to take a complete muscle-tendon complex out of the body and measure the force between its ends while it was active at different lengths, the final picture would be somewhat like that shown in Figure 3.2*b*.

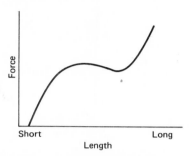

**FIGURE 3.2***b*. The effect of length change on force output in a complete anatomical muscle.

Our purpose here is to emphasize that the maximum force output that a muscle can produce is very dependent upon muscle length. Now we may not always want to generate maximum force, but even the same force will cost more in terms of metabolic energy if the muscle is in a disadvantageous part of its tension-length range. Surprisingly enough, we do not know exactly which part of the range described by the length axis in Figure 3.2*b* is what we might call the working range. The constraints of the joints of the body probably prevent us from using either extreme of this range but just how much of the middle part is used we can only guess.

## THE LEVERS OF THE SKELETON

Part of the reason that the tension-length properties of human muscle are not better known is that the properties of the isolated muscle are modified considerably when the muscle is put into its working position in the body—that is, linking together two bones on either side of a joint. Generally, muscles are only useful in that they produce a turning effect or moment about a joint. This turning effect is very dependent upon the angle between the bones of a joint. In Figure 3.3, part of a muscle called the biceps femoris situated on the back of the thigh has been schematically drawn. This muscle, which is one of the group known as the hamstrings, is joined to the thigh and

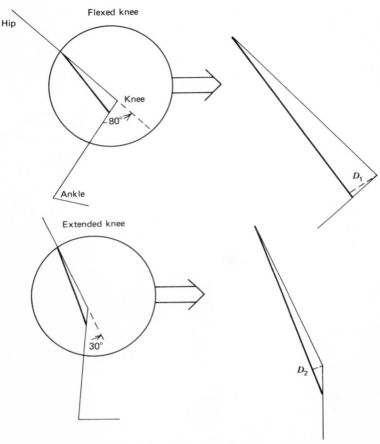

**FIGURE 3.3** The effect of joint angle on the turning effect that a muscle can produce. $D_1$ and $D_2$ are the moment arms in the two conditions.

shin bones (femur and tibia), and its task is to flex (bend) the knee joint. Now the turning effect of this, indeed of any muscle, is calculated as the product of the force and the moment arm, which is defined as the perpendicular distance of the muscle from the center of the joint. This distance is shown on the diagram as $D_1$ and $D_2$ for the flexed and extended knee, respectively.

If we assume that the muscle is producing the same force in the two

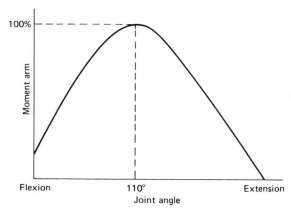

**FIGURE 3.4a.** The moment arm for the biceps femoris thoughout its range of movement. The largest moment arm (dotted line) is at a joint angle of about 110 degrees.

situations, the turning effect when the knee is flexed will be over four times greater because of the difference in perpendicular distance. Figure 3.4a gives a more precise picture of what the turning effect would be at various angles. The largest turning effect for any force would be at an angle of about 110 degrees, and this has been called 100 percent on the moment arm axis. Note how on each side of this optimum, what we might call the efficiency of the joint drops away. Now it is important that we consider both the effects of muscle length (Figure 3.2b) and leverage (Figure 3.4a) at the same time. They are both exerting their effects on the development of joint torque, and therefore these two graphs hold the secrets to understanding how the force that we can exert to a pedal will change throughout the range of joint motion. Remembering that when the joint angle is small the muscle is short, we note from a comparison of these two figures that, at small joint angles, in terms of both tension length and leverage, the muscle is at a disadvantage. This suggests that the combined musculo-skeletal system for knee flexion will be well below its optimum when the knee angle is small. At the other end of the spectrum, however, things are brighter. The effect of leverage is still bad news—we are past the optimum position—but now the tension-length curve is tending to compensate for the fall off that is due to leverage. We could describe the net result of these two factors as expressing the *competence* of a

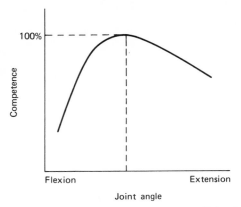

100%

Competence

Flexion                              Extension

Joint angle

**FIGURE 3.4b.** A theoretical "competence curve" for biceps femoris.
This graph combines the effects of tension-length and leverage to show the
relative competence of the joint-muscle combination at any joint angle.

joint to develop a turning effect. The competence curve for the knee
flexors is shown in Figure 3.4b, and you will see how the two inter-
acting factors have tended to give a plateau at greater joint angles.

Each muscle group has its own different competence curve for
every movement that the joint can make. For instance, knee extension,
which is a very important action in cycling, has an optimum competence angle in the region of 30 degrees, and the turning effect drops
off both above and below. We do have some control in cycling over
which part of the competence range a joint is working; adjusting the
seat height will clearly change this working range in all of the lower
limb joints and we will examine the experimental findings about optimum seat height in Section 7.

## MUSCLE ON THE MOVE

The effects of tension length and leverage that have just been described apply both when the joint is stationary, exerting an isometric
force, and when movement is occurring. However, during movement,
we must consider another important property of muscle known as the
force-velocity relationship. This property is fundamental to an understanding of why gearing is effective and concludes our description of
muscle in action.

When you are cycling along in a high gear and meet a gradient, as
your roadspeed becomes slower, you find yourself exerting very large

forces as the cranks turn over painfully slowly. Changing to a lower gear moves the cranks faster but the force applied is now smaller. Later we will consider what is happening to the force output at the wheel in these two situations, but our present concern is with the muscle. Most engines have a speed of operation at which they perform best, and skeletal muscle is no exception. The curve shown in Figure 3.5a gives an idea of what common sense has told us about our engine.

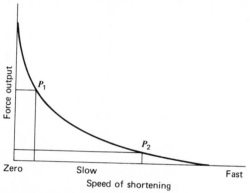

**FIGURE 3.5a.** The effects of velocity on the force output of muscle. The combinations of force and velocity shown at points $P_1$ and $P_2$ result in equal power outputs.

We can move large loads slowly and small loads fast. In the range of conditions shown in the figure, the largest force is when the velocity is zero—during isometric activity.

An interesting thing happens when we derive power output from this force-velocity curve. In Section 4 power is defined as work divided by time, but you will notice that the product of force and velocity has the same units as work/time and is indeed power. Graphically, the product is illustrated by taking any point on the graph (e.g., point $P_1$ on Figure 3.5a) and multiplying together the force and speed values that define the point.

It is clear that at the left and right extremes of Figure 3.5a, the power will be zero, since in one case velocity is zero and in the other, force is zero. The product of zero with anything is, of course, zero. This tells us that we have an optimum phenomenon. Somewhere between these two zero power points lies a combination of force and velocity at which peak power output can be derived from the muscle.

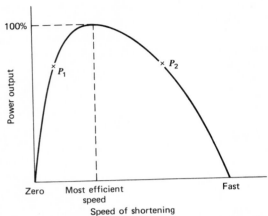

**FIGURE 3.5b.** The power output of muscle at various velocities. The points $P_1$ and $P_2$ correspond to those in part $a$ of this figure. The graph shows that there is a most efficient speed of shortening.

The whole power output curve has been calculated and drawn out in Figure 3.5b. The optimum conditions for this particular muscle occur when the force is about 35 percent of maximum isometric force with a corresponding velocity that is 25 percent of the theoretical maximum rate of shortening that the muscle can achieve. The concept of maximum rate of shortening is a little misleading, since it refers to the condition of zero load, which never occurs in the body. The curve, therefore, is not suggesting that slow pedalling rates are more efficient.

We should now be familiar with what gearing is all about. It is the process of adjusting the force exerted and the rate of shortening to move to a region of Figure 3.5b, which is as close as possible to the optimum point shown. Of course, you don't think of it in these terms when you are flicking through your available range to find the one that "feels best." If the effort is to be a long one, it is quite likely that the gear that feels best will be the one involving minimum energy expenditure and therefore maximum power output for each phase of activity.

As we will see in Part 2, there are many muscles involved in producing force output at the pedal, and each of them has its own tension-length and force-velocity curves. Thus the problem of fitting them all together is incredibly complex—so complex, in fact, that no one has ever tried to produce a mathematical model that would predict the most efficient conditions for pedalling from the data on the mechanical properties of muscle. What has been done though is to measure the energy cost of riding in different gears at the same speed and resistance. These experiments have confirmed that the principles outlined here do apply to movement of the whole body and underlie our need for gearing on a bicycle.

# PART II—THE MUSCLE OWNER'S MANUAL

The study of muscle so far in this section has been necessarily somewhat removed from cycling. It is now time to see how these fine pieces of engineering are arranged on the skeleton to produce forces that drive the pedals. We concentrate on the pelvis and lower limb, since these regions are most relevant for the cyclist. Our aim is not to turn the reader into an expert anatomist overnight, but instead, to give an overview of the system so that the major muscle masses can be identified and their role in force production outlined.

The framework to which the muscles are attached is shown in Figure 3.6. This is a scaffolding of over 30 bones for each lower limb. Let us take a pragmatic look at each of the major joints examining only the motion that occurs during pedalling and only the major muscles that are responsible for the motion.

## THE HIP JOINT AND A LOOK AT SOME GENERAL PRINCIPLES

The hip joint, between the head of the femur and the pelvis, is the best example of a ball and socket joint that the body has to offer. Since it has been estimated that the force being transmitted by the hip joint when a 150 pounds-force person is walking slowly can exceed 750 pounds-force, you can appreciate the requirements for strength. The socket is actually not as deep as you might imagine, but ligaments and muscles bind the joint together providing a very strong and stable system.

The movement of the hip joint that is most useful in cycling is hip extension (see Figure 3.7), but we must point out that the range of motion of the hip joint in cycling is quite unlike the motion encountered during other activities of daily life, with stair climbing being perhaps

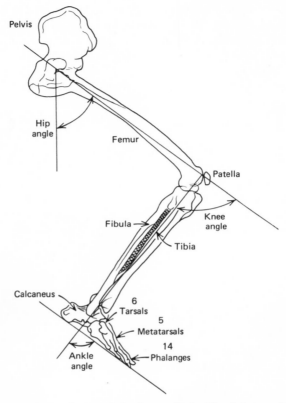

**FIGURE 3.6.** The skeleton of the lower limb. The joint angles shown are the conventions used to present the movements during cycling later in this chapter.

the closest approximation. Because the trunk leans forward and because of the geometric restrictions of cycling, the femur never actually goes behind the line of the trunk into what we would call an extended position. This is illustrated in Figure 3.8 where typical movements of all three major joints are shown both graphically and pictorially. All of these movements will of course be dependent upon seat height (see later chapter for more detail).

You will notice from the figure that a 30-degree hip angle is about the smallest recorded, and this represents the largest hip angle used in fast walking; so the ranges of motion for the two activities hardly over-

## Muscle Actions

| JOINT | FLEXION | | EXTENSION | |
|---|---|---|---|---|
| | One Joint | Two Joint | One Joint | Two Joint |
| Hip | 4 | 5 | 1 | 2 |
| Knee | 3 | 2 and 7 | 6 | 5 |
| Ankle | 8 and 9 | 7 | 10 | |

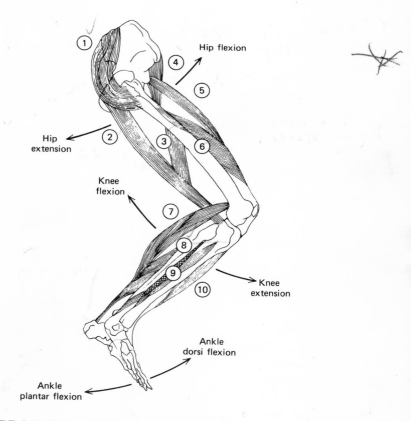

**FIGURE 3.7.** The major muscle groups of the lower limb used in cycling and a table of their actions.

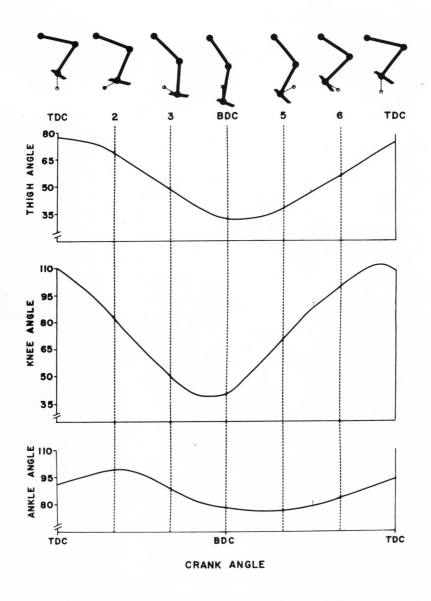

**FIGURE 3.8.** The movements of the lower limb in cycling above in pictorial form and below shown graphically.

lap. There is some evidence that strength training is specific to the joint angle at which training is performed. This means that if you are working on a weight-training program for cycling to improve hip extensor function, training at angles between 0 and 30 degrees will not have the benefit to your cycling that will accompany training between 30 and 80 degrees.

The major muscles producing hip extension are those labelled 1 and 2 in Figure 3.7—the gluteus maximus and part of the hamstring group. Together they form most of what is called the "hip extensor muscle group," and they introduce us to some concepts that will be a useful perspective on all the joints of the body. First, it is a general rule in the body, particularly in the limbs, that there are always two or more muscles that perform the same task at each joint. This is clearly useful where injury or birth defect puts one muscle from a particular group out of action but, in the healthy individual, it insures adequate strength throughout the full range of motion of a joint and makes possible some very subtle interactions between muscles.

The second major point to notice is that muscles can be ascribed to two distinct categories: those that cross only one joint and those that cross two or more joints. Most of the muscle groups that we examine have representatives from both categories and this is more than just an evolutionary accident. There are many situations where a two-joint muscle can perform two useful tasks much more efficiently than two separate muscles, one serving each joint, could do. However, there are several movements—and cycling has its fair share of these—where action of the two-joint muscles tends to produce movement at one of the joints that is the opposite of the movements required. In these situations there is a complex interaction between the one- and two-joint muscles, and the two-joint muscles definitely do not become inactive, despite their inappropriate action at one of the joints.

Looking again at the hip extensors, the gluteus maximus is the one-joint extensor and parts of the hamstring group are the two-joint extensors—crossing the knee joint as well as the hip. The gluteus is the familiar muscle—well-padded with fat—that forms the outline of the buttock. It is both extensive and important; human kind's development of erect posture has been associated, in part, with the development of this muscle. It is a large muscle, and the larger the cross-sectional area of a muscle, generally the more force it can produce. The gluteus maximus plays an important role in force production during cycling.

The hamstring muscle group is known to most of us, since we hear of people pulling or tearing hamstrings quite frequently. You can see from their location on the skeleton that when they shorten, they will tend to flex the knee joint as well as extend the hip. Look now at the joint actions in Figure 3.8, concentrating on the first half of the cycle where most of the propulsion is occurring. During the time when the hip is extending we note that the action of the knee joint is also extension. The hamstrings tend to flex the knee and if they are active during this period we will have encountered a case where the action of a two-joint muscle is opposite to the required motion at one of its joints.

## HOW CAN WE TELL WHEN MUSCLES ARE ACTIVE?

Knowing that a muscle is capable of performing a certain joint action is clearly very circumstantial evidence that it is actually active. The early anatomists—from the ancient Greeks until the decade of the 1930s—were only able to use palpation. They would lay their hand over a muscle and feel when it became hard during activity. You can try this yourself as you are riding along—put your hands over the quadriceps or hamstring group and try to feel when the muscle becomes active. You will find that it is very difficult to specify the exact position of the pedals when the muscle turned on and off, because the periods of activity are so brief.

Fortunately, because of the rapid developments in electronics in the last 40 years, we have the technique called electromyography (see Section 1), and this is a great help in pinning down the exact phasing of activity. Figure 3.9a shows a typical signal from the gluteus

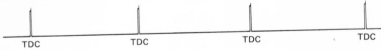

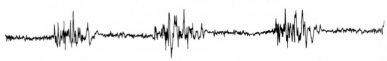

**FIGURE 3.9a.** Electromyograms of the gluteus maximus (muscle number 1 in Figure 5.7) during pedalling at 90 (revolutions per minute) TDC indicates Top Dead Center.

2 Analysize
i) Muscular
action.

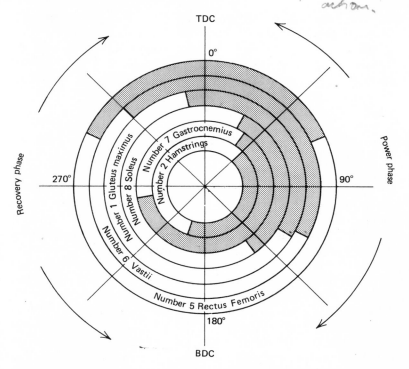

FIGURE 3.9b. The activity periods of six muscle groups during one revolution of the pedals.

maximus during a few seconds of pedalling at 90 revolutions per minute. When the muscle is not active the line is straight and parallel to the edge of the page but, as soon as activity begins, the ragged appearance of the signal tells us unequivocally that the muscle is working. We can treat electromyograms (EMGs) only as indicators of when the muscle was active and not, unfortunately, as an indicator of the force being developed. Let's return now to the hip joint and take the benefit of the fascinating insight that can be gained from EMGs.

You see from the figure that the gluteus maximus works for only very brief periods of time. It comes on with a short burst lasting about one-quarter of a second and is then silent for the rest of the revolution. Relating the activity to the position of the crank makes better visual sense and, in Figure 3.9b, this has been done for the gluteus maximus and five other muscles of the lower limb of a different subject. The

pedalling rate is again 90 revolutions per minute, and therefore a
45-degree sector is covered in less than one-tenth of a second. Look
at the sectors that represent the gluteus and hamstring muscles. We
see a trade-off occurring, with the gluteus maximus doing the first
45 degrees of hip extension on its own, and the hamstrings working
alone for the last 45 degrees; during the middle part both muscle
groups are active together.

Now the vastii muscles, which are the principal extensors of the
knee, are active at the same time as the hamstrings over a 70-degree
sector of crank movement. Therefore, we do have a case when, to do
their job at one joint, the hip, the hamstrings are generating turning
effects at another joint, the knee, that are contrary to the dominant
action. However, the final torque output at any joint represents the net
turning effect produced by both flexors and extensors, and therefore
we must assume that the knee flexors are producing a much greater
turning effect. The ways to regulate the turning effect are, as we have
seen earlier, by different lever lengths and different muscle forces, and
the delicate interplay of these two factors results in a smooth, coor-
dinated pedalling action.

Before leaving the hip joint we should mention the hip flexor muscle
group composed of muscles 4 and 5, the illiopsoas and the rectus
femoris, which are one- and two-joint muscles. These muscles are
partly responsible for the motion of the leg during the recovery phase.
Just what the illiopsoas is doing is largely a matter of guesswork,
because it lies so deep beneath other structures that we cannot easily
monitor its activity. The rectus femoris turns on during the last 90
degrees of the recovery phase (Figure 3.9b) when it could help to flex
the hip, but it also is generating force during the first 60 degrees of the
power phase. Again it is interesting to observe that, during this time, its
action at the hip is contrary to the dominant action—hip extension.

## THE KNEE JOINT

The knee and hip joints make strange neighbors; they are good
candidates for the most injury-prone and the most injury-free joints
in the body. The difference is that in the hip, there are bony parts of
the joint that withstand most of the external stresses but, in the knee
joint, soft tissue in the form of ligaments has to work with active
muscles to protect the joint to the best of their combined abilities. Of
course, what the knee is least equipped to cope with are the typical
football injuries where there is either a blow from the side or very

bad twisting; cyclists can be relatively sure that these kinds of situations are not going to arise in their sport.

One of the most interesting and useful features of the knee joint is a little oval disk of bone called the patella or knee cap, which slides along in a groove at the end of the femur. It is a member of a small group of "floating" bones that are attached at both ends to a tendon and have an articulation on one of their other surfaces. The function of the patella can be best understood by looking at Figure 3.7 while keeping in mind the discussion of leverage that centered around Figure 3.3. What happens is that the group labelled 5 and 6 on Figure 3.7—the knee extensors—have their efficiency radically improved by the presence of the patella. These muscles, the one-joint vastii group and the two-joint rectus femoris, together make up the quadriceps; all of these muscles terminate in the same tendon, which you can feel just above the knee cap when you tense the quadriceps. If the patella were absent this tendon would itself ride in the groove at the end of the femur on its way to insertion in the top of the tibia. The patella increases the turning effect of the quadriceps by moving the line of action of their combined force further from the center of rotation of the joint.

In contrast to the preponderance of one-joint extensors, most of the knee flexors are two-joint muscles, represented by muscle group number 2 in Figure 3.7. They attach to the pelvis and to the tibia with no attachment at all on the femur. The only one-joint flexor, muscle three in the figure, is again rather difficult to monitor and thus we concentrate on the most accessible muscles.

There is no doubt that knee extension is very important in cycling but there are some surprises in store when we look at the patterns of activity of the knee extensors in Figure 3.9b. The biggest surprise is that the vastii group are turned off when the crank is only 15 degrees past the horizontal while the knee flexors continue to act. This emphasizes that knee flexion and extension are both important in the production of force at different times in the pedal cycle—a fact that will be evident later when we examine direct measurements of forces applied to the pedal. It is worth pointing out here that many weight-training programs tend to ignore the knee flexors while working the knee extensors very hard indeed. The evidence that we have presented here suggests that cyclists planning a program to increase muscle strength must work with both flexors and extensors of the knee.

The recovery phase of the cycle where the knee and hip are both flexing is relatively devoid of activity in the muscles shown in Figure

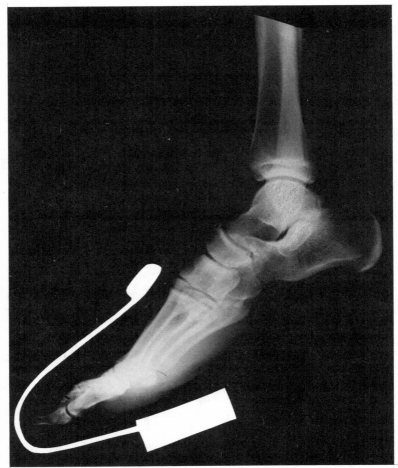

**FIGURE 3.10.** A medial X ray of the right foot with a typical position of the pedal and toeclip.

3.9*b*. This implies that the forces to move the limb are coming from somewhere else and we will discuss this possibility later.

## THE ANKLE AND FOOT

The integrity of the ankle and foot is dependent to a very large extent on ligaments; you can appreciate this by looking at the X ray of a right foot taken from the left side shown in Figure 3.10. The heel bone or calcaneus is not actually part of the ankle joint, although the major plantar flexors such as the gastrocnemius (muscle 7 in Figure 3.7) attach to it. The true ankle joint is between the bones of the leg and the small bone called the talus, which has a narrowing in the middle and sits on top of the calcaneus.

The position of the pedal has been drawn on the X ray, and all of the forces from the gastrocnemius, which will eventually reach the pedal, must be transmitted from bone to bone by the ligaments binding the tarsal bones together. This is completely different from the hip or knee where muscles act directly on the bones that provide the final force output. There are muscles attached directly to the metatarsal bones that are resting on the pedal, but the forces that these muscles can generate are many times smaller than those from the powerful gastrocnemius and soleus.

There is tremendous variation among healthy individuals in the flexibility of the ankle joint; at one extreme are the ballet dancers who can plantar flex such that the upper surface of the foot is parallel with the leg and, at the other end of the spectrum, are those who can neither point the toes or reduce the angle between leg and foot to much less than 90 degrees. An interesting consequence of the relatively small range of motion of the ankle joint is that the "competence" of the plantar flexors does not change a great deal because of leverage effects (see Part 1). For 30 degrees of movement on either side of the standing position (which is a large part of most people's range), the decrement due to leverage changes is only 13 percent in each direction.

It is difficult to categorize muscles acting about the ankle as one-and two-joint, as we have done with the other lower limb joints because, since no major muscles attach to the talus, all of the muscles cross more than one joint. This fact is usually ignored, and the soleus (muscle number 8) and gastrocnemius (muscle number 7) are usually called the one- and two-joint plantar flexors, respectively. It is interesting to note from Figure 3.9b that the gastrocnemius and soleus are turned on after both hip and knee extensors; the final link in the chain is the last one to be activated, but once it is switched on the gastrocnemius has the longest period of activity of any of the muscles shown in the figure. The actual movements of the ankle joint during cycling will be given special attention later, since they are a topic of special concern in pedalling style.

In concluding our discussion on anatomy, we don't want to leave you with the idea that the muscles of the limb are so well-distributed and distinct as the greatly simplified Figure 3.7 tends to suggest. Suppose for a moment that you were able to take a section through your upper

Front

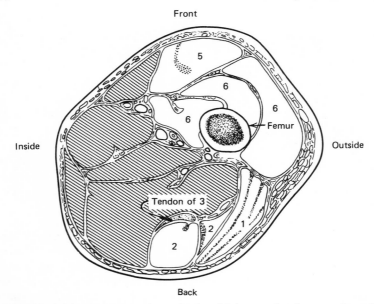

FIGURE 3.11. A section through the thigh at a level approximately 10 inches above the patella. The shaded areas are muscles that have not been mentioned in this section. Numbers correspond to the numbering system in Figure 3.7.

thigh. What would you see? Figure 3.11, which looks rather like a slice of lean ham, gives a good indication. The outline of the femur is apparent as well as some of the arteries, veins, and nerves that are in the section, together with the skin and fat surrounding everything. The shaded areas represent muscles we have not talked about, and the numbers correspond with those that we have. This should serve as a reminder that we have been rather specific in our coverage and there are many important muscle groups and joint movements that we have not mentioned.

## BIBLIOGRAPHY

Carlson, F. D., and D. R. Wilkie. *Muscle Physiology*. Prentice Hall, Englewood Cliffs, N. J. 1975.

James E. Crouch. *Functional Human Anatomy*. Lea and Febiger, Philadelphia. 1972.

# SECTION 4
# How Powerful Am I?

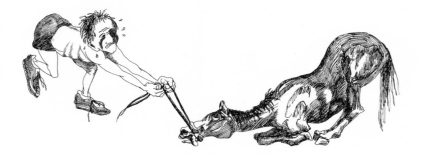

How powerful is your car, your lawnmower, or your kitchen mixer? How powerful are you—how powerful is a horse? Well, besides realizing that the last question is meant to make you say, "one horse power" (which paradoxically enough is incorrect), how many of the other points could you answer?

Before giving direct answers, we must backtrack a little and review some of the quantities that are used to define and quantify power. Let us begin with work; if you lift this book vertically through a distance of one foot, you have done a certain amount of mechanical work. Whether you raise it quickly or slowly the work done is the same as long as the distance remains the same. This is because work is the product of force and distance and is therefore independent of time. It is clear then that work is not the most useful indicator of performance in cycling; two cyclists climbing a hill would do the same amount of work despite the fact that one took only half the time of the other.

This discussion leads us directly to the definition of power. Power (more stricly, average power) is specified as work done divided by the time taken, and thus the first person to the top of the hill in the last example was developing twice the average power of the slower individual. The most widely used unit of power is the horsepower (hp)

51

which was defined by James Watt (of steam engine fame) rather arbitrarily to be one and one-half times the average power that a typical workhorse could sustain for a complete eight-hour day. The concept of power output being dependent upon the length of the work period is a crucial one, and we now explore this in more detail.

Imagine being asked to run as fast as possible up a long flight of steps, which was evenly divided into four sections. If your time over the first section was 15 seconds, it is a certain bet that on each of the next three sections the time would increase until you might be taking 35 seconds or more for the last exhausting part of the climb. Now, as we discussed earlier, since the work done in each section is the same, the power output must be decreasing as the time gets longer.

This change is characteristic of all "biological engines," and it has been the subject of some quite extensive studies. Figure 4.1 summarizes

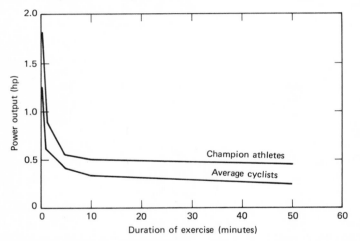

**FIGURE 4.1.** Maximum human power output for exersise of different duration. Data for champion athletes and average cyclists are shown. Adapted from Wilkie 1960.

what has been found to be the case during cycling for champion male athletes whose events lasted for the length of time shown along the bottom of the figure. A second curve for healthy adult males who were not athletes is also shown. First, look at the shape of the curves; you will see that power output falls very rapidly at the left-hand end but soon reaches a level that is almost steady; from that point onward, power output decreases only a small amount with large increases in the duration of exercise. Now look at the specific values of power output for the champion athletes; you will see that a sprinter, whose effort may be all over in 10 seconds, is developing between 1.5 to 2 horsepower, while champion athletes, who are working continuously for between 10 and 100 minutes, are able to continuously generate about 0.5 horsepower. Remember that these figures are for champion athletes working at or close to the limits of their performance. The maximum steady-state value (for exercise durations of 10 minutes or more) for the average individuals levels off at about 0.3 horsepower, and even this represents a much greater power output than most of us would care to maintain during touring or riding to the office. A figure around 0.1 horsepower is probably a more reasonable value for a nonexhaustive bicycle ride that lasts for an hour or so.

From Section 2, you will recall that the energy supply for short-duration work is almost exclusively *anaerobic*—that is, without oxygen. Indeed some sprinters hold their breath from start to finish, and it is anaerobic work that generages the highest power outputs. Once the work becomes *aerobic*—or completely fueled by oxidative metabolism—the power output is mainly limited by the capacity of the cardiovascular system to supply oxygen to the tissues. Since this is almost independent of work-period duration, we can see that the shape of Figure 4.1 makes some physiological sense.

So how do we compare with other engines? Well, unfortunately a small children's motorcycle with a capacity of 75 cubic centimeters can develop about 5 horsepower while a larger engine of 250 cubic centimeters is capable of 20-36 horsepower. Concerning your small kitchen mixer, it is likely to be capable of a power output of about 0.1 horsepower, therefore, though it might be a blow to our pride, we can place ourselves between a kitchen mixer and a toy motorcycle on the continuum of average power output!

The good news of course is that there are many redeeming features that makes the human engine, particularly the basic force element—skeletal muscle—extremely difficult to duplicate. It has been estimated that its thrust to weight ratio is an incredible 360, which is about 100 times better than a jet engine. Versatility is another key note that distinguishes human performance. Various specialized humans are capable of running 100 yards at average speeds in excess of 20 miles per hour riding 25 miles in one hour on a bicycle, lifting a weight in excess of 500 pounds overhead, running over 100 miles a day for days on end, or executing complex skills on the high bar in gymnastics. Our fuel sources are also very compact; to run a marathon the total fuel requirements weigh about 30 ounces compared to almost 10 pounds that one gallon of gasoline would weigh. Another critical difference is that our human engine can achieve vastly improved performance with training as we will see in Section 8. Having charted the limits of the human engine we can now proceed to investigate where and how the power of the engine is dissipated during cycling.

## POWER OUTPUT—A THEORETICAL EXAMPLE

We deal with the exact nature of the forces that are acting against the cyclist in the next two sections, but it is useful first to consider the situation shown in Figure 4.2. This example gives us the benefit of actually "seeing the enemy," which is certainly not the case with forces such as drag and friction that are encountered out on the road. The cyclist in Figure 4.2 is assumed to be riding on a level surface in a

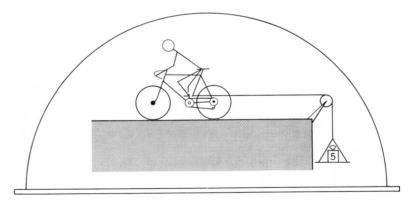

**FIGURE 4.2.** A theoretical situation where the only force slowing the rider down is the 5-pound weight that he is pulling up against gravity.

vacuum—therefore, there is no wind resistance (neither would he or she be able to breath, of course!) To extend the theory a little further, the bicycle is also assumed to be frictionless, the tires magically unresistive, and therefore, the only thing holding the cyclist back is the weight in tow, which can be varied by us to make the task easier or harder.

It is important to clarify the point that if the weight were carried on the bicycle or rider, the situation would be very different. This difference can be illustrated by the comparison of lifting a bucket of water from a well and then wheeling it on a frictionless cart. The first task (which is equivalent to our situation in Figure 4.2) would take considerable muscular work while the second would require a minimal power output.

Let's get back to the cycling example and begin with a weight of 5 pounds in the pan—equivalent to a single bag of sugar. Next, we must choose riding speeds, say 10 and 20 miles per hour, since we have made the point that power output is dependent upon the speed with which a task is performed. The power output can be calculated by the following formula:

$$\text{Power output} = \frac{\textit{Riding speed} \times \textit{Resistance}}{375}$$

When speed is in miles per hour and resistance is in pounds-force, the power output will be in the units with which we are now familiar—horsepower.

Now for the calculations: at 10 miles per hour the cyclist would have a power output of $10 \times 5/375$ or 0.13 horsepower, while at 25 miles per hour this would increase to 0.33 horsepower. When comparing these figures to the maximum values shown in Figure 4.1, we become aware of the surprising fact that at 20 miles per hour, this small resistance would require close to or above/maximum power output to overcome, and even at 10 miles per hour it requires more than what we might call a comfortable power output.

The real meaning of this finding is that particular care must be taken to identify and minimize the various forms of resistance in the actual riding situation. It is clear that the resisting forces need only be quite small to have a limiting effect on our capacity to ride at steady speeds. It is also fortunately true that any small reduction that we may cause in the resisting forces will have a considerable influence on our ability to ride more effectively. It is for this reason that we will spend the next two sections examining in some detail the four major "enemies" of the cyclist.

# BIBLIOGRAPHY

Wilkie D. R. "Man as a Source of Mechanical Power." *Ergonomics, 3,* No. 1, 1-8 (1960).

Whitt. F. R., and D. G. Wilson. Bicycling Science. Ergonomics and Mechanics. M. I. T. Press, Cambridge, Mass. Chapter 2.

Livingston C. L. "How Powerful Are You?" *Bicycling, 16,* No. 5, 46-47 (1975).

# SECTION 5
# What is Slowing Me Down?
# Hills and Tires

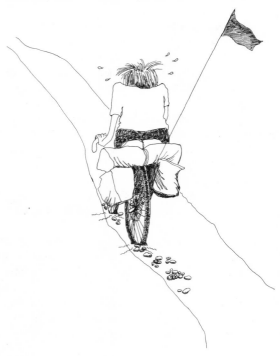

## HILLS

When we start cycling on the moon in our giant bubble containing a simulated earth's atmosphere, we will be disappointed to find that the level cycling will be no easier than it is here on earth, although steering will feel a little unusual. But when we come to the moon-hills, there will be some surprises in store! Climbing hills that we find impossibly steep on earth will be rather easy but, on the downhill stretches, it will seem to take us forever to pick up the speed we are accustomed to get from just coasting along. One of the important differences between the terrestrial and lunar environments is that the force of gravity is six times greater on earth than on the moon. You are probably thinking that this discussion is irrelevant, since there are enough problems getting bikeways constructed here on earth without looking ahead to moon navigation!

The comparison is a useful one, however, because it gives us some insight into the role that gravity plays in everyday cycling. It has been pointed out in the past that cycling is the most efficient form of animal locomotion on land. The major reason for this is that the body weight of the cyclist does not have to be supported against gravity by metabolic energy as it does in running and walking. As we will see later, gravity is indirectly responsible for some of the frictional forces but, for the moment, we ignore these. During level cycling the major effect of gravity is on the raising and lowering of the legs as they move during pedalling, and this is responsible for only a small part of the total energy expenditure.

It is difficult to give an exact figure for the energy cost of raising and lowering the limbs against gravity, since we also expend energy to rotate and accelerate the limbs, even though there is no resistance to pedalling. However, the total energy cost of doing all these things is only about 5 to 10 percent of your maximum output. It is possible to feel what this power output is like by taking the chain off, having someone hold your bike, and just spinning the cranks at a typical speed—say between 80 and 100 revolutions per minute. Although the skill takes a little while to acquire, it gives you an appreciation that some energy is spent just moving the limbs, even when you don't get anywhere.

Gravity has its most devastating effect when riding on hilly terrain as anyone who has pushed a heavily loaded touring bike up a steep hill and then hoped that the brakes would hold when coming down the other side can testify. To understand exactly why this happens we must relearn some of the findings that Galileo discovered almost 400 years ago. The following discussion is intended to give some understanding of how gravity acts on the cyclist.

A marble standing freely on an exactly level table will not move unless it is pushed. Of course, gravity is acting on the marble, but it is tending to pull it directly into the surface of the table. As soon as one side of the table is lifted slightly, the marble begins to roll. The force of gravity has not changed but it now has a component along the direction in which the marble is free to move.

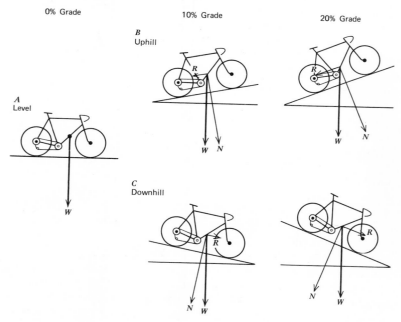

FIGURE 5.1. The effect of gravity on the level (*A*), and during uphill (*B*) and downhill riding (*C*) at gradients of 10 and 20 percent.

This is explained in Figure 5.1, where we see a cyclist on the level and on two hills of increasing severity. The force that is due to gravity is always the same, equal to the combined weight of the rider and bicycle, and it is always acting in the same direction, vertically downward. The other two arrows on the diagram have been obtained by a simple procedure called resolution of forces. This is something that you are very aware of intuitively but may not have formalized in the past. The force of gravity has been split up into two parts acting in new directions; the important thing is that the net effect of the two new forces will be exactly the same as the single force due to gravity.

We could have chosen to represent the force of gravity by forces in any direction as long as the net effect was always the same; but there is good reason to choose the directions shown in the figure, which you will note are parallel and at right angles to the road for the forces $R$ and $N$. The physical significance of the force $R$ is that it is exactly similar to the resisting force of the weight pan in our example of the previous section. It gives us an exact figure that can be used to estimate what the power output needed to climb hills of different gradients will be through the use of the formula, Power $= \dfrac{(\text{force} \times \text{speed})}{375}$

which was introduced in Section 4.

Examine the magnitude of the force component $R$ in the three conditions shown in Figure 5.1. On the level, it is equal to zero and therefore not shown on the diagram. The situation here is just like the marble on the level table. If the force of gravity were 10 times as great, the marble would still sit stubbornly in the same place because gravity does not have a component in the direction in which the marble is free to move. In the same way, this diagram confirms our earlier statement that on level ground, gravity is not very important in cycling. Since the force acting in the direction of progression is zero, our formula will predict zero power output against gravity at any speed.

On the hills, the situation is very different. The lines with arrows on them in Figure 5.1 are called vectors, and an important property of these lines is that they represent both the size of the force and the direction in which it acts. Now we know a typical value for the force $W$, which you will recall represents the combined weight of the rider and bicycle, might be 200 pounds. The size of the vector representing $R$ tells us that the forces opposing the cyclist's uphill motion are approximately 20 and 40 pounds-force in the two examples shown. These values are enormous when viewed in context of the 5-pound resisting force that was shown in Section 4 to require almost maximum power output at 20 miles per hour. It is this force component $R$, that becomes so limiting that we frequently decide to give up the fight, get off, and push or rest.

It is possible to do the calculation the other way around and, taking a given power output, predict what the maximum steady speed up these gradients would be. If the climber is given a maximum output of 0.35 horsepower (which, you will recall, will make it a pretty exhausting climb), these speeds turn out to be 6.6 and 3.3 miles per hour for the 10-percent and 20-percent grades, ignoring all other forms of resistance.

Before leaving the theory behind, there is one point that we have ignored: What happens on the downhill? Figure 5.1 shows clearly that on the same grade, the component $R$ is still the same size, but is now acting in favor of the cyclist. Another major way to produce forces in this direction is by pedalling, and the size and direction of the line $R$ in the downhill part of the figure is a quantitative expression of the relief we feel at the top of the hill when it is only necessary to sit back and hang onto the brakes. We will see in the next chapter how, despite the presence of the force $R$, which tends to continually accelerate the rider during downhill riding, a steady terminal speed is eventually reached because of the resistance of the air.

## WHAT CAN BE DONE ABOUT GRAVITY?

An "in joke" amongst biomechanists is about the high jumper who had a gravectomy—removal of his center of gravity—and was subsequently able to break all previous records. Unfortunately, gravity is unyielding to this and most other attempts to deny its influence, but there are various measures the cyclist can take that affect this particular enemy. Some of them are effective and beneficial in other ways while some are so insignificant as to be not worth the trouble.

One of the important things about $R$, the component of force due to gravity in Figure 5.1, is that its size is dependent upon $W$, the combined weight of rider and bicycle. This means, of course, that we have three options that will make hill climbing easier: we can lose weight off the bicycle, off our own body, or both.

Consider the weight of the bicycle first. Bikes come in all shapes and sizes with weights that vary from about 15 to 40 pounds-force. The low end of the scale represents the ultralightweight racing machine made from titanium or carbon fiber, while the heavyweights are the typical roadster machines made to last rather than to ride fast. It clearly makes sense to buy the lightest machine that will perform well under riding conditions that you typically subject it to. Each 1 percent saved in total weight, $W$, will result in a 1-percent reduction in the force component $R$. At small gradients this will represent quite a small value in actual pounds-force of resistance, but it becomes significant on steeper slopes. Also, at a given power output, the speed of riding and the resisting force are inversely related. What this means is that if you reduce the resisting force by a half, your speed will be twice as great, and not just 50 percent faster as a linear relationship would dictate.

However, we must remember that we are talking about 1 percent of the combined weight of the bicycle and rider. Therefore, although it may be possible through a bank loan or an unexpected windfall to purchase an ultralightweight bicycle, slashing the weight by 30 percent from 40 to 28 pounds-force, if the rider still weighs 160 pounds-force, the net reduction in the total weight is only about 5 percent. This 12-pounds-force weight loss from the bicycle that may have cost several hundred dollars would enable the rider in our previous example to make an average speed of about 7 miles per hour up a 10-percent grade rather than the 6.6 miles per hour previously possible (again, neglecting air resistance). This is a pretty expensive saving, and it reflects the fact that it is extremely difficult to do a great deal about the effects of gravity.

Before terminating this discussion on the effects of reducing machine weight, we should mention the enthusiastic cycling buff you may have encountered who has taken to attacking his or her bike with an electric drill. Indeed, drilling has recently become almost as popular a pastime with cyclists as it is with dentists. In the belief that the resulting reduction in machine weight will help the rider, chainwheels, handle bar extensions, and many other components have been honeycombed with holes. A liberal estimate of the weight saved by drilling 30 holes in a chainwheel is of the order of 1/2 ounce (14 grams). This would lead to a speed gain on a 10-percent grade of about 0.0014 miles per hour for a typical racing cyclist—or, in more understandable units, it would carry the cyclist three yards further during a solid hour of hill climbing. It should be clear from this calculation that drilling is a virtually useless way to improve speed or reduce energy cost on hills.

We have now reached the point of discussing weight loss in the other major component of the system—your body. You can probably guess the kind of advice we will offer in the following paragraphs. You are probably aware that you may be transporting considerable excess baggage in the form of body fat. Gravity makes no distinction between weight loss off the bicycle, which is bad for your checking account, and weight loss off the body, which may be extremely beneficial for your health in general.

A reduction in body weight will be reflected as a decrease in the force component, $R$, in exactly the same way as we have discussed for the reduction in machine weight. The moral is quite clear: before drilling or purchasing a new bicycle, consider whether or not you are overweight. If you are, then riding your bicycle a little more is a very good way to help your weight control while at the same time improving cardiovascular function and making hill climbing even easier than by weight reduction alone!

## SYSTEM MASS AND ACCELERATION

In our gravity dominated environment we have confused the relationship between mass and weight to the point where most people really do not know the difference. The bicycle and rider would still contain the same number of atoms whether gravity existed or not, and mass is a measure of this "quantity of matter." One of the most fundamental properties of matter is that of *Inertia*—the tendency to maintain the status quo. If a body is moving it tends to keep moving; if stationary, it will tend to remain there. This property is completely independent of gravity.

Most of the cycling situations that we have considered have involved steady-speed riding, and we must now briefly consider factors that affect acceleration and deceleration, which in city riding occupies a large part of a typical riding day. The reason for including this discussion here is that the acceleration characteristics depend on the mass of the bicycle and rider system, and the best way we have to judge mass is by weighing which really is looking at the effect of gravity. The more mass, the greater force there will be under an object and its support, because of gravity, and therefore we tend to use the concepts of weight and mass interchangeably in a loose manner, which would be unacceptable to the physicist.

As you know intuitively, and one of Newton's laws tell us explicitly, a heavier bicycle is very difficult to get up to speed from a standing start. The more mass in the bicycle the more its inertia—or, the more it resists a change of state. This change of state might be from rest to cruising speed, cruising speed to sprinting speed, or from sprinting speed to a complete stop. Since lightweight bicycles have more elaborate gearing, it is tempting to ascribe their livelier performance to the gears; however, gears are only a small part of it. Imagine an experiment in which 10-pound weights were loaded on the same bicycle and, after each increment of weight, the same rider was timed during a maximum effort from rest over a level, 25-yard course. If we give the rider enough time to recover between trials, there will be, within the limits of experimental error, quite a predictable relationship between weight added and time taken. The time taken will be approximately proportional to the square root of the mass; for example, a mass of 25 units would take 5 units of time while a mass of 36 units would take 6 units for the measured distance (this is of course total mass of bike and rider). Although this property is extremely important for racing cyclists who need to respond immediately to an opponent's move, it is not that crucial for the everyday pedaller. The concept of inertia is most meaningful for the average cyclist in the context of emergency braking.

A bicycle with more inertia (i.e., more mass determined by measuring more weight) will need a greater braking force to bring it to a halt from the same speed in the same distance. Therefore, the heavier bicycle will need to be equipped with better brakes, and the rider will need to be more wary of emergency situations. Fortunately, the effect of gravity on hills is so overwhelming that a bike heavy enough to give real problems in braking would be quite unrealistic to ride. Every time a small hill was encountered the rider would have to exert near maximal efforts, and the bike would be soon traded or sold.

In closing this discussion on inertia, we must mention the term, moment of inertia. This is the rotational equivalent of linear inertia that we have considered above. In this case, it is not only the quantity of matter that affects the resistance to change of state but also the distribution of the mass with respect to the axis of rotation. This concept can be nicely demonstrated by taking two front wheels of exactly the same type, two identical 1-pound weights, and some adhesive tape. Fix the wheels horizontally, and notice that it takes the same force to get the two wheels moving and to slow them down. Now tape the weights onto each wheel, putting one close in by the hub and the other at the tire. The wheel with the weight close in will feel about the same as before but the other wheel will need more force to get it spinning and will be noticeably harder to stop. Observe that both wheels, even with their weights taped on, have the same weight, but more weight is distributed further from the axis in one wheel leading to a greater moment of inertia. In fact, for the same additional mass, the moment of inertia varies as the square of the distance, and therefore if the weights were at 3 and 12 inches from the hub center, their moments of inertia about the axle were in the ratio of 1 to 16, respectively.

Using the same argument, it is true that lightweight rims will result in livelier performance, since a greater amount of inertia requires a greater torque (force applied at a distance from the axis) to produce the same acceleration. However, for most of us, a compromise weight and reliability has to be made. We need rims that will not be bent out of shape by riding over a pothole or drain grating. Generally, the heavier wheels will be more hardy—but, if acceleration is your requirement, then reduce the moment of inertia of the wheels together with weight on other parts of the bike.

## TIRES

Talking about wheels leads us nicely to the next in our list of energy absorbing enemies, rolling resistance. You can feel the effects of this form of resistance by reducing your tire pressures until they are just above the safe limit (i.e., without damaging the tires) and see how difficult it is to climb a hill that you would normally have no trouble with. Rolling resistance actually depends upon more than just tire pressure, and those who are technically minded will find a good description of the phenomenum in Whitt and Wilson. The principal idea is that even with a steel wheel running on a steel surface— a railway engine wheel and track—the materials are never quite rigid enough for there to be a single point of contact between the two surfaces. Therefore, in an exaggerated case, it is like riding on "square wheels" where the point of contact between the wheel and road is forward of the wheel center for much of the revolution. The analogy is not quite strict enough however since, as the bicycle wheel rolls, the same total area of the tire and road remain in contact. It is clear that the greater the area of this "patch" of tire and road that are in contact, the greater the resistance will be, since the contact region will extend further in front of the wheel center. With the same wheel, tire, inflation pressure, and road surface, the area of contact will be a function of the loading on the wheel. This form of resistance is therefore also dependent upon gravity to some extent. It is for this reason that the units of rolling resistance are the somewhat unusual pound-force per pound-force, the first unit being the resistance to rolling in pounds of force and the second being the vertical loading on the wheel.

The four most important factors that affect rolling resistance are wheel diameter, road surface, tire type, and inflation pressure. For cylinders on plane surfaces, the rolling resistance is inversely proportional to the radius of the cylinder. This means that small-wheel bicycles will have more resistance to motion than large wheels under the same conditions. It is significant that the popularity of these small-wheel diameter bicycles has been limited to the "about-town" kind of activity where the fact that the bike will fit easily into the trunk of a car is a more important consideration than any other.

Road surface has a considerable effect on rolling resistance as participants in cyclo-cross will readily agree. Riding on soft sand or gravel is often so strenuous as to be limiting and, in this extreme case, the rolling resistance can exceed the available force output of the cyclist. Each road surface will offer a different resistance to a given wheel; more experimental work has been done on this topic using automobile wheels than with bicycles, and data from these studies indicate that there is, for example, approximately a 5-percent difference between the rolling resistance of concrete and blacktop.

The two factors influencing rolling resistance over which the cyclist has most control are tire type and inflation pressure, and a manipulation of both of these can influence rolling resistance considerably. Experiments performed for the Schwinn Bicycle Company give important insight into the effect of these two variables upon rolling resistance on a standard road surface. Table 5.1 shows data from six tires running at their recommended inflation pressures on the same surface. The rolling resistance coefficient is shown together with the actual retarding force for a 180-pound rider and bicycle combination.

We can see from this table that it matters very much which tire you choose, since the resistance to motion varies dramatically over a threefold range, meaning that the worst tire will abosrb three times more of your metabolic energy than the best one. The equation developed in Section 4 for power output indicates that the two extreme tires would require power outputs of 0.14 and 0.04 horsepower at 15 miles per hour ignoring all other forms of resistance.

The real breakpoint comes when you switch from what are known in the United States as "clinchers" to "sew-ups." Clinchers, the standard tire, have a wire insert around their inner circumference; they need a separate tube and rims that have a "U" section. Sew-ups are a self-contained tire and tube unit. There is no wire rim, since the tube is sewn inside the tire, which is then glued onto a rim of almost rectangular cross section. The operating pressure of the sew-up tires is generally at least 30 to 40 pounds per square inch greater than the clincher, and this will cause a slightly rougher ride.

If you have never tried sew-ups and feel you can afford them, you have a pleasant surprise in store. The lower rolling resistances shown in Table 5.1 for the sew-ups are very noticeable indeed and will make

**TABLE 5.1** Effect of tire type on rolling resistance

| TIRE TYPE | INFLATION PRESSURE (psi)[a] | COEFFICIENT OF ROLLING RESISTANCE (lbf/lbf)[b] | ACTUAL RESISTANCE (lbf) |
|---|---|---|---|
| Breeze* | 65 | 0.0190 | 3.42 |
| Puff* | 75 | 0.0091 | 1.63 |
| Clement (Road No. 50) | 105 | 0.0070 | 1.26 |
| Letour (National) | 105 | 0.0067 | 1.21 |
| Clement (Road No. 13) | 105 | 0.0058 | 1.04 |
| Clement (Track No. 3) | 105 | 0.0056 | 1.01 |

[a] Abbreviation for pound-force per square inch.
[b] Abbreviation for pound-force.
*These tires are clinchers.
All others are sew-ups

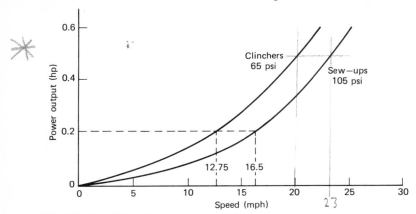

FIGURE 5.2. The effect of using either clinchers or sew-ups on riding speed at various power outputs. At 0.2 horsepower the increase in speed would be almost 4 miles per hour if sew-ups were used.
(From R. D. Rowland and R. S. Rice, Calspan Technical Report # ZS-5157-K-1. April 1973.)

your cycling easier or faster depending upon your objectives. The difference is shown graphically in Figure 5.2, where the speeds on both tires can be determined, assuming the rider puts out the same amount of power. The dashed horizontal line shows a power output of 0.2 horsepower. With given conditions of weight, frontal area, and zero gradient, this power output would result in a speed of 12.75 miles per hour with clinchers. A substantial increase in speed to 16.5 miles per hour would be obtained simply by switching to sew-up tires. For the average rider, the choice of tires is equally critical as it is for the racing cyclist, and perhaps even more so. This is because rolling resistance can influence power output more than drag at low riding speeds in still air.

To switch to sew-ups from clinchers will, of course, mean investing in a new set of wheels, because of the different rims, and it will also result in some maintenance costs. Sew-ups are very much more accident prone; you may have seen cyclists who use sew-ups carrying a spare in their back pocket or tucked under the saddle. Since the flat is usually thrown away, keeping mobile can be an expensive proposition. Also, since the rims are less sturdy, the compromise between optimum performance and durability mentioned earlier must be made to suit each individual rider.

Although it is extremely unlikely that a clincher tire would be used

**TABLE 5.2** Effect of inflation pressure on rolling resistance

| TIRE | INFLATION PRESSURE (psi) | COEFICIENT OF ROLLING RESISTANCE (lbf/lbf) | INCREASE IN ROLLING RESISTAN FROM 105 psi |
|---|---|---|---|
| National | 85 | 0.0076 | 13.43% |
| Road No. 13 | 85 | 0.0064 | 10.34% |
| Track No. 3 | 85 | 0.0063 | 12.50% |

by a racing cyclist, it is interesting to note that there is a variation of
about 20 percent in the resistance offered by different tires that the
racing cyclist might use. It is a case of there being insufficient data to
make a choice of tire based completely upon published quantitative
data. Also, there are many other factors to be considered such as
traction under various weather conditions. Hopefully, concern expressed by cyclists will encourage manufacturers to make more data
available in the future to allow a meaningful comparison of different
tires. In many cases the manufacturer knows the values for rolling
resistance of various tires and is simply choosing not to let the customer
know.

## THE EFFECT OF TIRE PRESSURE

Tire inflation pressures have a major effect on rolling resistance.
Table 5.2 shows the effect of reducing inflation pressures for two of
the tires considered in Table 5.1 and a track tire. It is clear from the
table that a 20-pound per square inch reduction in inflation pressure
increases the rolling resistance by approximately 12 percent in the tires
considered. Although no data for lower pressures are currently available, it is likely that the resistance increases nonlinearly with further
decreases in inflation pressures.

It is astonishing how little attention the average rider pays to cor-
rectly inflated tires. Too often the signal to do something about inflation is when the rim bumps the road surface. Not only does this increase rolling resistance dramatically, and damage tubes and tires,
but also it can be dangerous, in that maneuverability is adversely affected.

In summary, rolling resistance can affect your cycling considerably
if you use clincher tires or you do not keep your tires inflated to the
correct pressures. With both of these factors corrected, it can be reduced to a plateau level that does not vary appreciably with speed,
and thus its percentage contribution to the total resistance actually
reduces with speed, since drag becomes more important at higher
speeds (see Section 6).

## BIBLIOGRAPHY

Tricker, R. A. R., and Tricker, B. J. K. *The Science of Movement.*
American Elsevier, New York. Chapters 6, 7 and 8.

Whitt F. R., and Wilson D. G. *Bicycling Science: Ergonomics and
Mechanics.* M. I. T. Press, Cambridge, Mass. Chapter 6.

# SECTION 6

# What is Still Slowing Me Down? Drag and Friction

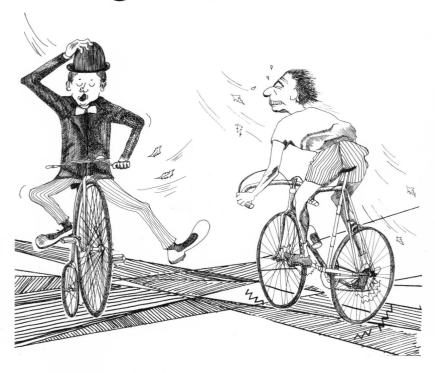

It was estimated in a recent article that during a ride of 100 miles, the cyclist pushes aside 9636 pounds of air. Every cyclist should know that the manner in which this air is pushed out of the way will have an important bearing on the total energy expenditure. World speed records for a bicycle made behind cars or motorcycles equipped with large windshields are in excess of 100 miles per hour. When this is contrasted with the unpaced, unshielded speeds of approximately 30 miles per hour during a 1000-meter flying start on the track, the critical importance of this form of resistance becomes apparent. An understanding of the origin of air resistance and measures that can be taken to minimize its effect would clearly be of benefit to the cyclist.

Although we don't see the air in front of us on level ground, it is the single most important factor that limits cycling speed. What makes drag (or air resistance) a most sinister enemy is that it can constantly change its force. The exact nature of the changes are rather complex but there are some general rules, derived both from theory and experiments, that will be useful to know.

Once we fix the physical characteristics of the cyclist and bicycle, the most important determinant of drag is relative cycling speed. Relative speed takes into account both riding speed and windspeed, and it is therefore the same at 10 miles per hour riding into a 15-mile per hour headwind as it is cycling in still air at 25 miles per hour. The change in drag with speed is an interesting one, and Table 6.1 shows the drag force at various relative speeds (ignore the lower part of the table for the moment). Notice how at speeds below 10 miles per hour, the force is rather small but, as relative speed increases, it rises very rapidly. By 25 miles per hour, the resistance has risen to over 5 pounds of force, and we have seen in earlier sections that this will require a power output that is beyond the capacity of most of us.

**TABLE 6.1** Variation in drag and power output with speed of cycling

| Speed (mph) | 0 | 5 | 10 | 15 | 20 | 25 | 30 |
|---|---|---|---|---|---|---|---|
| $(\text{Speed})^2$ | 0 | 25 | 100 | 225 | 400 | 625 | 900 |
| Drag (lbf) | 0 | 0.21 | 0.86 | 1.93 | 3.43 | 5.36 | 7.72 |
| $(\text{Speed})^3$ | 0 | 125 | 1000 | 3375 | 8000 | 15625 | 27000 |
| Power (hp) Output | 0 | 0.002 | 0.022 | 0.07 | 0.18 | 0.35 | 0.61 |

It may not be news to you that you cannot ride 25 miles in one hour but neither of course, can you ride 10 miles in one hour if there is a headwind approaching 15 miles per hour and this seems a little more relevant. The rapid increase in drag with relative speed is what is known as a direct square relationship. The drag is actually proportional to the square of the relative speed. Notice the second line in Table 6.1. This is the square of the speed, and the size of this number gives an indication of the magnitude of the drag relative to the drag at 1 mile per hour.

Those readers anxious to use their electronic calculators will by now have divided the values for drag given in line 3 by the values for speed squared in line 2. Each time they will have got an answer close to 0.0086. What this means is that at any speed, the drag force can be calculated as follows:

Drag in lbf = 0.0086 × (relative speed in mph)$^2$

The 0.0086 is a constant that includes assumed values for the effects of size, shape, and environmental conditions, and we touch briefly on some of these shortly. If the fact that drag increases as the square of speed is bad news, there is even worse to come! The way to calculate the power output to overcome a given resistive force was given in Section 4. It is the product of force and relative speed. In the current context, this means that power output is proportional to the cube of speed.

Look now at the second half of Table 6.1—here you see the cube of speed ($v^3$) and the power output in horsepower. The numbers now are enormous and tell us that 2000 times the power is required to overcome drag at 20 miles per hour than at 1 mile per hour. At 30 miles per hour the factor is a staggering 27,000 times, and this requires power outputs that are all but impossible for the average person.

Here we stress that the problem of drag is not a simple one. Consider, for instance, the following question: What would happen to the ground speed of a cyclist pedalling in still air at 20 miles per hour who suddenly encounters a 10-mile per hour headwind without changing his or her power output? Most people make a first response that the ground speed would be 10 miles per hour, which is wrong, because of the direct cube relation between power output and relative speed. The actual answer, 14.1, miles per hour, is obtained from solving a cubic equation and is clearly divergent from the first guess.

Before we introduce some experimental findings that will be of use to you, we must briefly discuss the effects of winds that are not simple headwinds. In general, they will approach the cyclist obliquely and, to calculate their effect, we must use vector addition. This procedure produces one resultant vector from two or more components and thus is the reverse of resolution of vectors that we met in Section 5.

Figure 6.1 is a vectorial representation of riding due north at 10 miles per hour against an 8-mile per hour wind coming out of the northwest.

The effect of travelling 10 miles per hour under any condition is, of course, to generate a headwind of 10 miles per hour, and this vector must be combined with that for actual wind. The resultant can be described geometrically as the diagonal of the parallelogram of which the two contributing vectors form adjacent sides. Mathematical formulation or a graphical analysis enables us to predict a relative wind-speed of 16.6 miles per hour coming from 20 degrees west of north.

It is instructive to carry this calculation two stages further. First, we make the assumption that the cyclist and bicycle are the same shape when viewed from every direction—rather like a travelling cylinder. We know this assumption is incorrect but it will do for the moment. The drag felt by the cyclist can now be calculated from our previous discussions, and this will be 2.4 pounds-force in the same direction as the resultant wind velocity.

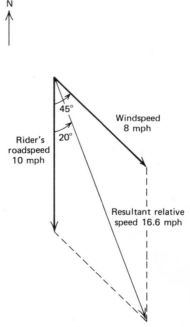

**FIGURE 6.1a.** Calculation of relative speed by vector addition of roadspeed and windspeed.

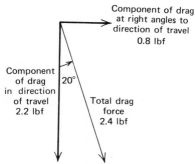

**FIGURE 6.1b.** Resolution of drag force into two components. Note that the arithmetic sum of the components does not equal the total, since we are dealing with vectors.

Now the final step is shown in Figure 4.1b. Drag itself is a vector quantity, and it can be resolved into two components in any direction, for example, south and east. Only the component directly opposing the cyclist, the force of 2.2 pounds-force due south will directly affect power output. We know all about that because it is now the same as a force produced by a headwind. But what about the force of 0.8 pounds-force, which tends to accelerate the cyclist in a direction 90 degrees away from the intended course? The force will have to be equalized by side forces from the tires and a slight lean "into the wind" that will cause a gravitational component to act. This position, particularly with a large drag force acting laterally, looks extremely unlikely when photographed from behind, but it is part of the series of subconscious riding skills that we have carried with us from the early days of learning to ride.

There are two misconceptions concerning the effect of wind that we should dispel at this point. The first one is that on a closed-loop course, the work done battling against wind on the outward journey will be completely balanced by the benefit obtained from the wind when returning. Unfortunately, this supposition is not true—again because of the direct cube relationship between power output and cycling speed. We can expand on this a little from an article by Livingstone (see end of Section) who showed that there is always a wind direction that will produce fastest times on a given closed-loop course. He gave a sample calculation of time variations of over 2.5 percent for a racing cyclist expending 0.4 horsepower on a 35-mile triangular course with the wind coming successively from all points of the compass. This difference may seem small, but bicycle races are often won or lost by one-tenth of a second, and in a time trial the contestants start at different times, which means that different cyclists may encounter different winds.

The second misconception is the statement that winds in the sector from due west through south to due east will help the northbound cyclist, and those from the semicircle in front of the cyclist will be harmful. This apparently sensible argument is not borne out by calculations. Another example from the same article is the case of a northbound racer with a power output of 0.4 horsepower. The surprising fact is that a wind will only be assistive for 164 of the 360 degrees of the possible circle of directions. It is beyond the present scope to go into details of the mathematics but is worth remembering that the wind is not necessarily as friendly as you might imagine.

Enough of the theory. What can you do to reduce the effects of drag or at least to live with it in the most comfortable way? The most obvious, almost reflexive, thing to do when meeting a wind is to crouch over the handle bars. What exactly is achieved by doing this? Well, one of the most important of the several things buried in our constant of 0.0086 is a figure for the frontal area of the cyclist and bicycle. You can conceptualize the meaning of frontal area if you imagine posing in front of a screen and looking at your shadow cast by bright parallel light. The larger the area of the shadow, the more drag force will be felt. It has been estimated that, for an average person, the typical upright, touring, and racing positions have frontal areas of 5.4, 4.5 and 3.7 square feet.

Drag force is directly related to frontal area; therefore, if we change riding positions from the upright to the crouched racing position, reducing the area by 30 percent, the drag force will also be reduced by 30 percent. The best illustration of these effects is seen in Figure 6.2. Along the horizontal axis, this figure shows the speed of riding under the "base" conditions of level riding in the touring position in still air. If at this speed the rider crouched down, the speed gain can be found by moving vertically until the upper line is met and then moving horizontally to read off the value for speed gain from the vertical axis. Similarly, if the rider changed from the touring to the upright position, the speed loss can be found by moving down to the lower line and again finding the appropriate point on the vertical axis.

Now, suppose two cyclists were riding at 15 miles per hour in the touring position and one assumed the upright position the other the

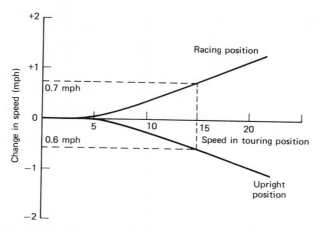

**FIGURE 6.2.** The effect of changing position on roadspeed assumng the power output remains the same. The dashed line shows that at 15 miles per hour, changing from the touring position to the racing position would increase speed by 0.7 miles per hour while sitting upright would decrease speed by 0.6 miles per hour.
(From R. D. Rowland and R. S. Rice. Calspan Technical Report # ZS-5157-K-1. April 1973.)

racing position—neither changing their steady power output. The dotted lines on Figure 6.2 represent this condition and show that the speed of the "croucher" would increase by 0.7 miles per hour and that of the "upright sitter" would decrease by 0.6 miles per hour, making their new speeds 15.7 and 14.4 miles per hour, respectively.

We should mention here that a touring position is one in which the rider's hands are on the top of the handlebars or resting on the top of the brake levers. The racing position is the full crouch where the rider grasps the bottom of the dropped handlebars and tries to get as low as comfort will allow. The upright position is not really possible on a ten-speed machine without loosing the handlebars, but it is common on the older "sit up and beg" machines with handlebars that bend straight back toward the rider.

The values in Figure 6.2 are from theoretical predictions—they are the output of a simple mathematical model. Considering the overwhelming importance of drag to cycling, it is amazing that there are only isolated examples in the literature of direct experiments on the effects of drag. One of the few studies to date where cyclists have been put in a wind tunnel (see Section 1) was carried out in England in 1956. It produced some very interesting results, despite its limited scope—only three male cyclists were used.

First, the bicycle is, as you might guess, a very messy structure aerodynamically. When the bicycle was put in the tunnel by itself, the drag force recorded was approximately 30 percent of the force recorded when the rider was sitting on the bike. The actual drag caused by the bike is probably less when the rider is shrouding parts of it. Now the racing cyclist is bound by the rules of the sport to make no modifications to the basic structure of the bicycle that will enhance the aerodynamic capabilities. The rest of us can do just what we like, and it is strange that some enterprising manufacturer has not produced a bike with a few aerodynamic modifications. Chester Kyle (see references at end of the section) has been a pioneer in this respect, and he has shown that by simply stretching a plastic sheet between the frame members, and using a similar sheet to partly shield the wheels, the drag of the bicycle was reduced by almost 50 percent. Disc wheels

Concerning changing position on the bike, the wind tunnel experiments confimed the predictions of improvements to be gained by crouching in a racing style. However, a further stage was possible where once the rider had adopted the customary crouching position, the experimenter asked him to make small modifications such as tucking the elbows in or changing the position of the head. The wind was then switched on, and a measurement was made to determine the effectiveness of the change in posture. The results were fascinating.

With one rider, small modifications were made and these reduced the drag force by 5 percent. Exactly the same modifications in a second rider who was slightly lighter and shorter actually increased the drag. The results with this powerful technique show clearly how individual the fine tuning is to produce the best aerodynamic shape. Drag is as important to skiers as it is to cyclists, and recently members of several national ski teams have been put in wind tunnels and encouraged to experiment with a variety of small adjustments to their "egg-shaped," downhill posture until the very best configurations were found.

We have not really dealt with the question of shape but you have certainly been wondering about it—we are all used to seeing such beautiful aerodynamic shapes as the nose of the Concorde or a formula 1 racing car. The shape of an object is generally more important than frontal area as a determinant of drag, and a glance at Figure 6.3 should

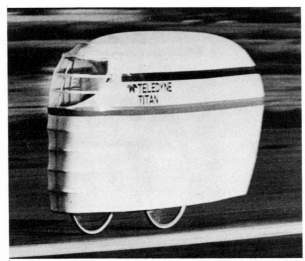

**FIGURE 6.3.** A steamlined fairing in the shape of an aircraft wing mounted on a bicycle that was riden at speeds of over 40 miles per hour.

convince you of this. Despite appearances, what you see in the figure is a bike, but the structure built around it was designed by Chester Kyle to change the shape presented to the air. On a level course, this machine, when powered by a champion cyclist, has reached sprint speeds of 43 miles per hour and averaged over 40 miles per hour for a mile course. It is rather unstable and very susceptible to crosswinds but is nevertheless a testimony to the importance of shape, especially since the frontal area is considerably greater than a regular bike and rider.

While we are talking of speed records, you may be interested to know that the current record for a one-hour ride on a standard bicycle was set by Eddie Merckx in Mexico City. This venue was carefully planned because of air density, another factor hidden in our constant of 0.0086. The density of the air does, of course, vary at the same location from day to day but it varies most with increase in elevation. At higher altitudes, the air is less dense, and consequently the force due to drag is less. It is not surprising then that a potential world-record holder planned to make use of every slight advantage available. Clearly the reduction in drag force outweighed the lower oxygen content that would have made sustained exercise slightly more difficult.

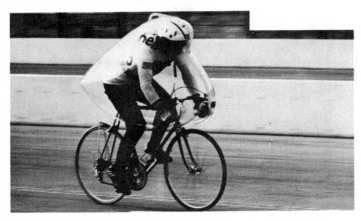

**FIGURE 6.4.** A fairing designed to provide a better shape to the air flow and to be relatively easy to use. This device would need extra care in the presence of side winds or high speed traffic.

Another recent innovation aimed at a more general audience and designed to improve shape is the fairing shown in Figure 6.4. This transparent, plastic device fits over the head, trunk, and arms of the rider and offers considerably improved aerodynamic characteristics. As with the complete fairing, extreme care must be taken particularly when gusty side winds are likely. The penalty for reduced frontal drag is increased drag to side winds, which could result in uncontrollable changes in the rider's direction.

Although it is impractical to build a bicycle like the one in Figure 6.3 for everyday use, there are some very practical things the rider can do to reduce the effects of drag. The first of these is to choose clothing wisely. An interesting test was done in the wind tunnel experiments mentioned earlier. One rider, who had been wearing a racing jersey and shorts for the other experiments, put on street clothes that included a jacket and long trousers. When measurements were taken in the wind tunnel it was found that the drag force increased by an astonishing 30 percent.

Flapping trouser legs and jackets that act as wind socks are very costly in terms of the energy needed to overcome additional drag force. When deciding which clothes to wear for bike riding, these experiments give us some very clear instructions: choose those that offer the least amount of additional frills that the wind can get hold of. Of course, the clothes must not be so tight fitting that they restrict the movement needed to pedal but, apart from this, the tighter they fit the better.

A second important way to reduce drag is to let someone or something else do most of the work against the air for you. I am almost ashamed to admit to a favorite pastime of my friends and me in high-school days. We would follow the school bus travelling at 30 to 40 miles per hour for several miles at a distance of 12 to 18 inches while our girlfriends gazed admiringly from the backseat. Our girlfriends didn't know much about drag and therefore looked on our feat as close to superhuman. (The bus driver, however, knew a lot about safety and finally ended our escapades.)

What we were doing was "drafting," and the most celebrated example of this in cycling is the four-man team pursuit. In this Olympic event, a team of four riders follow each other in a line, often with only inches separating their wheels. While the rider at the front is "breaking the wind," his or her teammates are able to recover until the time comes for their turn at the front. The dramatic way the front rider peels off up the banking and the need for skillful precision riding makes this one of competitive cycling's most spectacular events.

The reduction in drag force that can be achieved by following another rider closely is very considerable. There have been some fascinating experiments with both runners and cyclists to document the exact gains, showing for example that even at a speed of 15 miles per hour, the fourth cyclist back in a tightly packed line uses only about three-quarters of the power of the leader. These experiments suggest that the best strategy for a group of recreational riders on a windy day is to continually alternate the lead, allowing each rider to gradually move up the line as the first rider moves to the back and is able to recover.

Finally concerning drag, we will talk briefly about the concept of terminal velocity. When freewheeling down a long hill you are probably aware that you eventually reach a steady speed. Exactly the same thing happens to a free-fall parachutist; after the initial acceleration a steady "terminal speed" is reached, even without the parachute being open. In both these instances, we are seeing an exact matching of the forces of drag and gravity. The force due to gravity ($R$ in Figure 5.1) is the same at all points on a hill of uniform slope. However, at the top of the hill when the rider is just picking up speed, the drag force, although in the opposite direction, is small and the net result of these two opposing forces still tends to accelerate the cyclist. Eventually, as speed is increased, the force due to drag (which we know rises rapidly) approaches the value of the gravity component. At this point there is no net force on the rider who therefore continues at a steady speed. This is an interesting example of a battle between a fixed force and a variable one.

It is instructive and indeed frustrating to coast down hills with a rider who is heavier than oneself. Without a good deal of pedalling from the lightweight individual, the heavier individual soon disappears into the distance. It is also a good chance to experiment with the effects of shape and frontal area to see if the heavier rider, by sitting upright, can slow down to the speed of the lighter person who is adopting a posture more like a racing cyclist.

## FRICTION

It is certainly true to say that without friction there would be no cycling as we know it. Riding in a frictionless world would be like a combination of riding in a vacuum, on ice, with wet rims. Turning would be lethal, and stopping would be impossible. It is clear then that there are many situations in which friction works to our advantage, particularly in traction and braking, and we examine some of these. There are, however, several sources of friction that cause excess energy to be expended. Obvious sources are poorly lubricated, worn, or badly adjusted components. Because of this dual role of friction, we are going to depart from the format of considering only the forces that retard the cyclist for a more general view of friction.

Let us begin by drawing a distinction between two basically different kinds of friction. Consider the situation where you are standing beside your bike and applying a gentle pressure to the front brake. At the same time, you start to push on the bike as if to move it forward. At first nothing happens but, as the force tending to advance the bike becomes greater, movement eventually occurs.

The force tending to push the bicycle rim past the brake blocks was, in the premovement stages, less than a critical value known as the limiting frictional force. At every stage until movement occurred the frictional force changed its value to become just great enough to prevent movement. If, at the critical moment when slipping first occurred, we could measure the force with which the bike was being pushed forward and the force the brake blocks were applying to the rim, the ratio (forward force/brake-block force) would give us a value called the coefficient of static friction—given the symbol $\mu_s$ (pronounced, mew sub $s$). We examine this in more detail in a moment.

We continue with the experiment a little further. The bike has begun to move and, while still applying the same pressure to the brake lever, we find that the force needed to keep the bike moving at a constant speed is considerably less than what was needed to initiate movement. We have rediscovered the fact that the coefficient of gliding or kinetic friction (called $\mu_k$, pronounced mew sub $k$) is much less than the coefficient of static friction for the same surfaces under the same conditions. (The calculation for $\mu_k$ is [steady forward force/ brake-block force]). In other words, we have found that it is hard to start two surfaces slipping over each other but, once the slipping has started, it is relatively easy to keep the slipping going. This is clearly good news for the rider who is not yet in a skid but bad news for the rider already skidding.

## STATIC FRICTION

The most important example of static friction in cycling is the traction between the rear wheel and the road. This is clearly an example where the propelling force must be less than the limiting frictional force or the wheel will spin aimlessly. The cyclist does have a considerable amount of control over the limiting frictional force between bike and road, as we show in Figure 6.5. The force $B$ represents the reaction force under the back wheel, and it is changed by the position of the cyclist on the bike. For example, it might be 80 pounds-force when the rider is leaning forward and 140 pounds-force when he or she is sitting back. The limiting frictional force can be calculated, as shown in the figure, by multiplying $\mu_s$ by this reaction force. Taking a typical value for $\mu_s$ of 0.8, we find that forces of 64 and 112 pounds-force could be exerted by the tire on the road before slipping would occur in the forward and sitting-back positions.

A quick look forward to Section 7 will indicate that forces at the tire of this magnitude are extremely unlikely. It would take a pedal force of over 600 pounds-force to produce these propulsive forces in a typical gear. So we can conclude that, under the conditions specified, spinning of the back wheel is very unlikely.

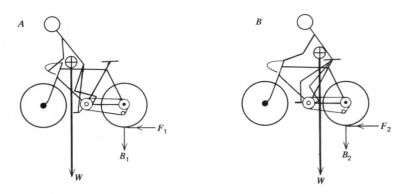

**FIGURE 6.5.** The change in (the limiting) frictional force between rear tire and road as a result of the rider changing position on the bike. The calculation is explained in the text.

We are not finished with this topic yet because, as we know, road and weather conditions change and what that means in mechanical terms is that $\mu_s$ changes. In fact, in wet weather, the coefficient of friction may be reduced by up to 10 times and by much more under icy conditions. Consequently, the limiting frictional forces in Figure 6.5 will also be reduced by a factor of 10 or more, leading to maximum forces at the tire of 6.4 and 11.2 pounds-force before slipping occurs in the two positions. These kinds of forces are very possible, requiring pedal forces of only 36 and 63 pounds-force. Now the advantage of shifting the weight becomes clear. In wet or icy weather, moving off the seat to apply more force to the pedals may be self-defeating, since the amount of force tolerated at the tire/road interface before slipping occurs will be reduced.

The problem in wet weather is that a thin film of water interposes between tire and road in just the same way as lubricating oil keeps the metal-bearing surfaces apart. Many people feel that tread patterns on tires are for the purpose of increasing $\mu_s$ under dry conditions. This is not the case. They allow the water to be squeezed out from under the contact area into the grooves of the tread pattern. For car tires, the tread patterns are essential but, at the low speeds generally used on bicycles, it has been suggested that fancy tread patterns do very little indeed to prevent slipping in wet weather.

# FRICTION AND CORNERING

Slipping of the back wheel as a result of pedalling forces, while irritating, is not generally dangerous. The kind of slipping that occurs in cornering—where the bicycle glides out from under the rider—is potentially very dangerous, and we consider briefly the mechanics surrounding such events.

When we turn a corner there is a force, known as a centrifugal or centripetal force, which is trying to accelerate us out of the turn along the line joining bike and the center of the turning circle. The force is countered by leaning into the turn to produce a turning moment in the opposite direction using the force of gravity. The faster we attempt to take the turn the larger the centrifugal force is, and consequently the more lean is required. What the lean actually does is to ensure that the cyclist does not "fall out of the turn"—that is, fall away from the center of the turning circle. It does not change the fact that there is a horizontal force tending to make the tire slip away from the center of the turning circle, and this force must be less than the limiting frictional force for a nonslip condition.

For each curve there is a critical speed that must not be exceeded if skidding is to be prevented. Some simple calculations show that the safety margin is quite wide, and indeed most cyclists can judge what is an unsafe speed under normal conditions. The problem comes with conditions that are not predictable; in mechanical terms, the coefficient of friction changes at various points on the turn. Gravel or water lying in patches on the road are capable of changing the coefficient of friction by a factor of 10. The safe speed is a function of the square root of the coefficient of friction. Therefore, if the coefficient drops by a factor of 9, the safe speed will drop by a factor of 3. Riders must realize that there are additional forces when turning, and they must be aware that friction is the only thing between them and a meeting with the road—and friction may leave just when they need it most!

# DYNAMIC FRICTION

A useful grouping in our discussion of dynamic friction is that which is useful and that which is not. A leading contender for the most useful site of dynamic friction is in bicycle brakes. Brakes could be called energy converters, since they convert the kinetic energy of motion into heat with the help of muscular energy from the hand or leg. They are almost always operating in the region where the force driving the rim through the brake blocks is greater than the limiting frictional force. The relevant coefficient is therefore the coefficient of sliding or kinetic friction, $\mu_k$, and you will recall that this is generally less than the static coefficient.

Unfortunately, $\mu_k$ modifies its value under wet conditions in a similar manner to $\mu_s$. This change is much more lethal on a bike than in an automobile, since the brakes are exposed, and any water that is cleared during the first few revolutions of the wheel is likely to be quickly replaced.

Experiments conducted at M.I.T. have shown that a wet wheel will turn an average of 30 times with the brakes full on before an appreciable increase in the coefficient of friction occurs. It will then take another 20 revolutions until values comparable with dry surfaces are obtained. In practical terms this means that in the worst case on a regular bike with 27-inch diameter wheels, you may have travelled a startling 350 feet past the reason for wanting to stop before you get the best response from your brakes. The moral in this tale is that bike brakes are just not designed for wet weather; extreme care and reduction in riding speed are indicated wherever there is water on the road.

For a complete coverage of braking, refer to Whitt and Wilson, *Bicycling Science.* We only mention a few major points here. When braking is underway the reaction force under the rear wheel (*B* in Figure 6.5) is considerably reduced, even when the rider is sitting back in the saddle. This means that the limiting frictional force between the tire and road is also reduced, and it will be easy to lock the back brakes and start skidding. There is much more braking power available in the front brakes because of the increased reaction force between front tire and road—so much in fact that care must be taken to insure that the rider does not exit over the handlebars.

It is surprising that the frictional force applied by brakes does not vary with the area of contact. Thus, if the brake blocks were only half as long, the initial braking force would be the same. Since friction generates heat, the performance of brakes really depends on how much heat they can dissipate, and this is a function of brake-block area. Smaller brake blocks would therefore heat up and undergo "fade"— a reduction in the coefficient of friction with a consequent reduction in braking efficiency. The tread pattern on brake blocks does help with wet weather braking to some extent but, as we mentioned earlier, as far as brakes are concerned wet weather means danger.

## THE HOT SEAT

One of the most noticeable places that friction is present is between the saddle and the areas of skin on the rider overlying those bony parts of the seat—the ischial tuberosities. We return to this topic in Sections 7 and 12; at this stage we note that if there is excessive movement or inadequate interface between rider and saddle, the tissue in the area will become inflamed from heat generated by the frictional forces. This is certainly the first and the most uncomfortable in our series of undesirable sites for friction, and we discuss how to deal with this problem later.

## FRICTION IN THE MACHINERY OF THE BIKE

The time has now come to lay what blame we can on friction for slowing us down in the same way that we tried to estimate the effects of gravity, rolling resistance, and drag. On a well-adjusted bike, we can make the general statement that friction consumes very little of our metabolic energy. It is theoretically possible to derive an overall coefficient of friction for the whole bike. In practice this proves a little difficult, particularly when trying to partition the effects of rolling resistance out of the measurements. Most authorities will not be pinned down to an exact estimate of the power losses that are due to friction, but place it at much less than 5 percent.

However, this estimate could increase dramatically as a result of poor maintenance and particularly poor adjustment of the bicycle. For example, a fender or carrier stay rubbing against the tire is a very effective friction brake, as is a poorly aligned or buckled rear wheel that may cause the tire to rub against the frame. A significant loss of power may result from poorly adjusted brakes that rub against the rim at some point in the revolution of the wheel.

The nature of the bicycle transmission is such that some power is dissipated in heat as a result of friction, though this is considerably less than the power lost in an automobile transmission. A greater loss is associated with hub gears than derailleur gears, since in the former several trains of meshing gear wheels inside the hub are used to produce the required reduction, each carrying the penalty of power loss. The chain is an important element in the system and must be kept clean and watched for signs of wear or stretching, which will increase friction. Friction of moving parts on the bike is therefore only a minor enemy of the cyclist, provided that good attention has been paid to lubrication and maintenance.

## BIBLIOGRAPHY

Lambie, Jack, "Catch the Wind." *Bike World, 3,* 10, 20-22 (1974).

Kyle, Chester. "What Affects Bicycle Speed." *Bicycling*, 22-24 (July 1974) and 28-29 (August 1974).

Livingstone, C. L. "Beating the Wind." *Bicycling*, 58-61 (July 1975).

Whitt, F. R., and D. G. Wilson. "Bicycling Science." Chapters 5, 7, and 8.

# SECTION 7
# How Do I Pedal?

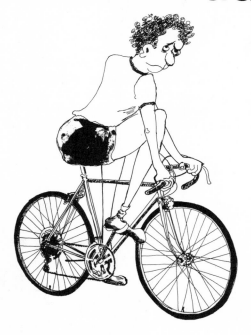

Cycling is somewhat unique among sport movements in that at least one part of the body is constrained to move along a predetermined path. This does not mean, however, that the individual is left without the choice of how to move certain joints. In the simplest model, the lower limb is composed of three rigid segments, freely jointed at the interconnections. Even if the ends of such a three-link chain are moved along specific paths, the motion of the segments are still indeterminate, in other words, there are an infinite number of possible movement patterns. However, anatomical restraints remove certain of the possibilities and, if seat height is taken into account, the similarities in the patterns of joint movement chosen by skilled cyclists are more striking than the differences. Here we discuss how force is applied to the pedals, how that force is in turn applied to the road, and we look at both the opinion and the evidence on how such important factors as seat height and ankle action should be determined.

Looking at the motion of the limbs, as we did in the section on muscle action, does not tell us anything about the forces that are being produced to drive the bicycle. To get this information we have to devise some special equipment and, as long ago as 1889, an ingenious scientist called R. P. Scott made the first force-measuring pedal, which was fitted to the large wheeled "ordinary bicycle" of the day. While Scott's equipment was obviously not as sophisticated as what is available today, he nevertheless made some observations that still have relevance. Several more recent studies in which the author has been involved have made use of the force and angle measuring pedal shown in Figure 7.1. The following description is a synthesis of the available research evidence.

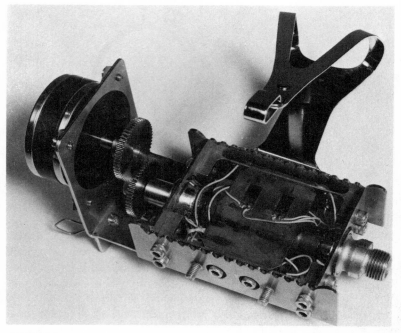

FIGURE 7.1 A pedal designed at Penn State University to measure forces and pedal orientation during cycling.

How do you think you pedal? Do you push steadily throughout the first quarter or the first half of the revolution, do you pull up on the backstroke, do you push more with one leg than the other? If you are anything like the subjects that we have studied in the laboratory, your own perception of your pedalling pattern is not necessarily an accurate one, so let's look at some actual patterns.

Although it may feel to you like a steady force, chances are, if you are a reasonably good cyclist, that your pattern of force application is something like that shown pictorially in Figure 7.2. In this diagram

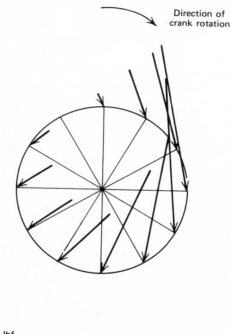

FIGURE 7.2. The size and orientation of the force applied to the right pedal by five racing cyclists working at about 60 percent of their maximum and spinning at 90.

(From R. J. Gregor, Ph.D. Dissertation, Penn State University, 1976.)

the size of the arrow indicates the size of the force, and the orientation shows the direction in which the force is applied. The scale indicates that the largest forces are of the order of 60 pounds-force. There are several points of interest in the diagram. First, notice that the subjects were exerting very small forces as the pedal came over what we call top dead center (TDC) and the forces rose progressively throughout the first quadrant. The maximum value is usually reached at about 120 degrees—that is, 30 degrees past the horizontal. Next, notice how the arrow is pointing forward at the top of the power stroke and pointing back by the bottom of the stroke. Finally, note that there were still forces with a downward component during the recovery part of the cycle. I should add that these patterns are the mean from five racing cyclists who were wearing toe clips. The work load was such that the cyclists had to use about 50 to 60 percent of their maximal oxygen uptake to continue pedalling at the required rate of 90 revolutions per minute. Let us discuss some of these observations in more detail and see just what they imply for your pedalling action.

## IT'S THE TORQUE THAT COUNTS

If you only carry away one idea with you from this chapter, let it be this one: you may be exerting a larger force on the pedal than any known cyclist before you but, unless the force is in the right direction, it will not necessarily result in large propulsive forces at the wheel. "Simple," you might say, but look at the torque or turning effect that several forces produce. In Figure 7.3 we see the crank in a position of 30 degrees past the vertical and four forces, all of the same magnitude, but in different directions. Alongside the diagram you will see an indication of how effective the force is in producing torque. It may surprise you to see that the vertical force that would result from a straight push down is the least effective of all the forces shown in this position of the crank.

The degree of effectiveness will, of course, vary as the crank angle varies; for example, the force $F_1$ would have zero effectiveness at top dead center and bottom dead center but would become 100 percent effective halfway through the power stroke. There are two ways to find how effective any force will be: either you can resolve the force into two components, one at right angles to the crank and one parallel to the crank, or you can find the moment arm—the perpendicular distance of the line of action of the force from the center of the crank axis.

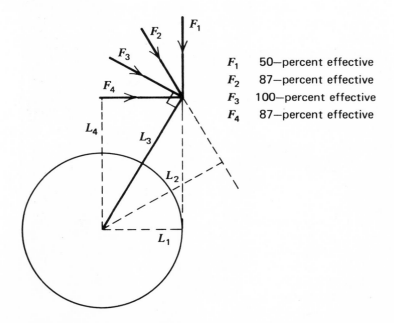

| | |
|---|---|
| $F_1$ | 50—percent effective |
| $F_2$ | 87—percent effective |
| $F_3$ | 100—percent effective |
| $F_4$ | 87—percent effective |

**FIGURE 7.3.** The effectiveness of the same force applied to the pedal at four different angles. The moment arm of each force about the crank is drawn ($L_1$, etc). Note that a simple vertical force is the least effective of all the conditions shown.

This last approach is a little easier to explain graphically; the moment arm for each force has been shown on the diagram ($L_1$, $L_2$, etc) and, if you measure them up, you will find they are in the ratio of the effectiveness values shown in the figure.

For metabolically efficient cycling it is important that large forces are not applied in directions that produce small turning effects. Looking back to Figure 7.2, we see that this rule was followed fairly well by the cyclists studied for the first quarter of the revolution. There was only a small force at TDC and, as the crank moved through the quadrant, an effort was made to orient the force at an angle that was more advantageous than a simple vertical push. In the second quandrant it seems to have become difficult anatomically to give the force vector an optimal orientation and, although the vector goes past the vertical, the force being exerted at bottom dead center is only about 15 percent effective.

It is very interesting to note what happens during the recovery phase shown in Figure 7.2. The force on the pedal never falls to zero, even though the subjects were wearing toe clips and cleated shoes. If the subjects had been actively pulling up on the pedal, the arrows would indicate upward forces but you see that they never do. Several experiments have confirmed that in relatively moderate riding situations, toe clips appear to be useful simply because they keep the foot in the correct position on the pedal. Many unfounded statements such as: "toe clips virtually double pedalling efficiency" can be found in cycling books. The evidence shown in Figure 7.2 would certainly appear to contradict these kinds of statements. It is likely that in more taxing situations, such as hill climbing, the toe clips are used to exert upward forces but the exact amount of benefit they give still remains to be determined.

The downward and rearward pointing arrows during the recovery phase in Figure 7.2 should be considered carefully. Part of this force is what might be called a "lazy leg action." Remember that we are only seeing the output from one leg in the figure and, during this time, the opposite leg is in its power phase. What is happening then is that the opposite leg is having to push some of the weight of the recovery leg before the forces that it is exerting can be usefully applied to the wheel. Also contributing to the forces shown are the dynamics of the recovery limb. The limb segments involved are being accelerated in a direction opposite to that of the arrows, and muscle action may be undesirable at this time.

We cannot yet say if this is a good or bad feature of the pedalling action but certainly, if there were very large downward forces being exerted by the recovery leg, it would represent considerable inefficiency. The major point here is that at this work load, there is no direct evidence of pulling up on the clips that were worn by all five cyclists whose average pedalling patterns make up the figure. This would tend to suggest that, under these conditions, the clips help maintain the position of the foot on the pedal and little else.

It is possible to combine the data on pedalling forces from both legs and come up with a torque curve that is shown in Figure 7.4.

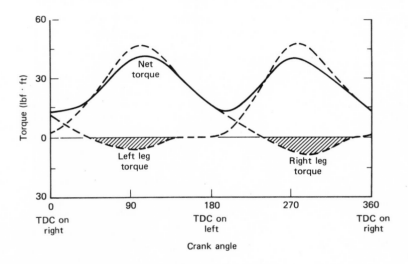

FIGURE 7.4. The net torque on the cranks during a complete revolution of the pedals. The torque developed by the left and right legs separately are shown in dotted lines, and where these are negative the counterproductive areas have been shaded.

This curve from the same five cyclists shows the mean pattern of the effective parts of the applied forces from both legs during one complete pedalling cycle. Figure 7.4 is the really important one as far as propulsion goes, and an exact reflection of this curve is what will appear at the wheel. It is far from a steady output, as you can see, and represents the final summation and interaction of all the muscle forces, their anatomical levers, the angle of application of the forces to the pedal, the ankle angle, in fact, almost all of the biomechanical factors that we have discussed up until now. The individual curves from each leg separately have been included as dotted lines and, where the torques are negative, that is, counterproductive, they have been shaded.

The net curve has smaller peaks than the two individual ones, but you will see also that the net torque is never negative because one leg is always producing a larger positive torque at times when the other leg is generating negative torques.

It may come as a surprise to you that even during apparently steady cycling, the torque output falls to 30 percent of its peak value at the low points that are just past TDC for each crank. Indeed these patterns are from relatively skilled racing cyclists and, unless you pay careful attention to style, your patterns may be even more ragged.

## THE QUESTION OF SYMMETRY

Several years ago we did some experiments to determine how much work was done with each leg during pedalling on a laboratory bicycle. Although we didn't expect the results to be exactly 50 percent for the left and 50 percent for the right, what we actually found was quite a shock. The curves shown in Figure 7.4 seem to be quite symmetrical but a few of the riders in this study who thought that they were pedalling with an even balance between left and right legs were really doing almost twice as much work with one leg than with the other. Smaller amounts of asymmetry were quite common. These were all healthy young individuals who rode a bike to get around campus. An even more confusing occurence was that when we brought the subjects back on another day, we found that they may have had no asymmetry, the same asymmetry, or completely opposite asymmetry, and therefore we could not relate the observed differences to limb dominance.

There are two possibilities for what might be happening here-: first, a cyclist may make a subconscious decision which limb is going to be the dominant one on a given day. Second, during a bout of riding, there may be constant changing between one limb and the other—while one limb does more than its share of the work the other limb rests. We could not distinguish between these two hypotheses in our experiments, since the pedalling periods were too short.

The results of these experiments carry the implications that most of us who ride bikes do so, to some extent, asymmetrically. Taken to extremes, this imbalance could result in early fatigue in the muscles of the extremity doing most of the work and must be considered to be inefficient pedalling. Correction of the fault will clearly be difficult if the perception of an asymmetric action by the cyclist is inadequate. It may well be of value during training rides for the cyclist to deliberately overemphasize the action of each leg for a period of time to become more aware of what asymmetry feels like. Also, during "off the bike" training sessions, efforts should be made to exercise both legs; weight training is particularly useful here, since the limbs can be both tested and trained individually.

### FROM PEDAL TO WHEEL

Most of our discussions of forces and torques have stopped at the crank axis and, before getting to seat height and ankle action, we should consider briefly the transmission of forces through the bike to the road. Figure 7.5 really tells the story for us. In the figure, a 50-

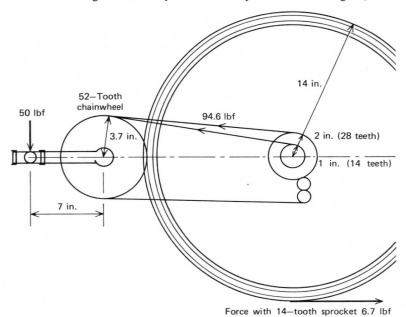

Force with 14—tooth sprocket 6.7 lbf
Force with 28—tooth sprocket 13.5 lbf

**FIGURE 7.5.** Force at the tire in two different gears when a steady force of 50 pounds-force is exerted at the pedal in a direction that results in 100 percent efficiency.

pound force is being exerted on the pedal at an angle that results in a 100 percent effective turning effect. The example uses two-gear combinations; both have a 52-tooth chainwheel, but rear sprockets of 14 and 28 teeth are shown. The small sprocket is an example of a high gear, since one revolution of the pedals would move the bike 100 inches, while the second gear would be a low gear with 50 inches of forward movement for one pedal cycle.

Both gears result in a force of 94.6 pounds in the upper length of the chain but, by the time we get out to the circumference of the driving wheel, the useful force output is 6.7 pounds for the high gear and 13.5 pounds for the low gear. Make sure you have these forces the right way around. The lower gear gives greater force at the wheel for the same pedal force. The penalty for the low gear is, of course, that the pedals are moving faster, and high pedal forces are just not possible at these rapid rates because of the force-velocity considerations discussed earlier. Also, the fast pedal speeds (above 120 revolutions per minute) rapidly become physiologically inefficient at high road speeds.

Your first thought on seeing these wheel forces is probably that they are surprisingly small—even ridiculously small—and that the author must have got his arithmetic wrong. You can, however, convince yourself that I am correct by standing your bike upside down and, while pressing down on the pedals with one hand, stop the back wheel moving by holding onto the tire with the other hand. You will be surprised at how little force it takes to stop the wheel from moving, despite the effort you are applying to the pedal. The ratios of wheel to pedal forces for the examples we have considered would be 1 to 7.5 and 1 to 3.7 for the high and low gears, respectively.

There is another relevant comparison here; turn back briefly to the sections on the forces that slow the cyclist down, and you will see that their magnitudes are similar to the wheel forces that we have calculated here, For example, the drag force at 15 miles per hour when riding into a 10-mile an hour wind is just over 5 pounds, and the force due to gravity for a 200-pound rider and bike is 20 pounds on a 10 percent grade. Therefore the 50-pound pedal force would be sufficient to overcome the wind only in the lower gear but neither gear would allow the rider to climb the hill without an increase in pedal force.

There is one important difference between the forces at the wheel and the resistive forces such as gravity and drag. The resistive forces offer a steady, unchanging pull, trying to slow the cyclist down and ac-celerate him or her in their direction. However, the wheel forces will be a direct, scaled-down version of the net torque curve that we found from Figure 7.4. to be anything but constant. What must happen then is that the average wheel forces must be at least equal to the sum of the steady opposing forces. Of course there are times, such as on undulating terrain or in a gusty wind, when it is an oversimplification to treat the opposing forces as steady, but in general they will be far more constant than the torque output.

## WHAT IS THE CORRECT SEAT HEIGHT FOR YOU?

When you move the seat post an innocent inch or two up or down, you are changing the action of virtually every muscle in the lower limb that is involved in the pedalling action. This adjustment, if it happens to be the wrong one, could be extremely costly in terms of energy de-mands, and the whole procedure therefore deserves careful exam-ination.

Imagine for the moment that the seat adjustment on your bike is by some coincidence, at the very best height for you—a position that we will define shortly. If we were able to bring you into the lab and measure your oxygen uptake at this seat height and at two others—one slightly higher and one slightly lower—we would be able to demon-strate one of the many "optimal" phenomena that occur in the body. Both conditions that were away from the best height would need more oxygen to sustain the same work load—giving a "U" shape to the curve of oxygen uptake against seat height. Some of the other "optimal" phenomena include a most efficient speed of walking (expressed as energy used per unit distance), a minimal oxygen uptake per unit dis-tance as downhill gradient is varied during running, and of course an optimal gear ratio for each cycling speed.

The reason why this optimal point is reached has been documented in the section on muscle action. The change in seat height changes the range of joint angles that are used to pedal, and this in turn puts the various muscles at different points on their tension-length curves. The  angular velocities of the joints also change, and muscles move from the most efficient range of their force-velocity curves. The result for the cyclist is that more oxygen must be consumed, and the work becomes harder than it really should be—causing a drop in efficiency.

The drop in efficiency is usually less than 10 percent for heights that most people might try, and it appears to be more if the seat is too high than if it is too low. It would be a mistake to interpret this evidence as suggesting that it is safer to have the seat too low than too high. Oxygen uptake is only one of the factors to consider; when the seat height is very low it is likely that the forces tending to dislocate the knee joint are increased considerably. Pain and possible injury far outweigh the benefit of erring on the side of efficiency.

Experiments have been carried out where the seat height has been varied over a wide range in the same individual and oxygen uptake is used to define the optimum seat height for that person. The results have led to a convenient method for getting the seat adjustment into the region right for you. While standing upright in shoes, you should have someone take your inside leg measurement from crotch to floor, just as if you were being measured for a pair of trousers. The distance between pedal surface and the top of the saddle measured along the seat tube should be set to 109 percent of the inside leg measurement. The measurement is illustrated in Figure 7.6, and Table 7.1 will enable

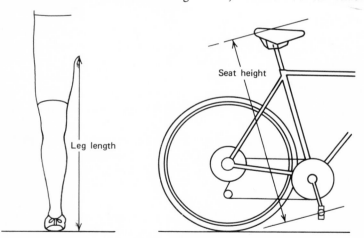

**FIGURE 7.6.** Measurements required to determine the correct seat height for your leg length. (a) Inside leg length is taken from crotch to floor. (b) Distance marked SH on the figure is set to 109 percent of leg length value. See Table 7.1 for sample distances.

you to find the correct measurement for your leg length. Note that the seat height given in this table is not from the floor to the seat but from seat to pedal, as shown in Figure 7.6.

**TABLE 7.1** Reasonable seat height for your leg length (See Figure 7.6 for details of the measurements)

| Inside Leg Length (in.) | 26 | 27 | 28 | 29 | 30 | 31 | 32 | 33 | 34 | 35 | 36 |
|---|---|---|---|---|---|---|---|---|---|---|---|
| Seat Height (in.) | 28.3 | 29.4 | 30.5 | 31.6 | 32.7 | 33.8 | 34.9 | 36 | 37.1 | 38.1 | 39.2 |

To get an idea of what this seat height looks like in action, four shots of the lower limbs of a subject riding at close to optimum seat height are shown in Figure 7.7. The angles that the limbs are moving through are close to those described in the earlier section on muscle action. A higher seat height would need more knee extension at the bottom of the stroke, while a seat height that is too low would result in the exaggerated knee lift exhibited by the cartoon character on the introductory page of this section.

A final word about seat height; do not treat the formula given here as a rigid rule that you must get used to even if it continues to cause you agony. By all means experiment. The best way to go about the experiment is to use the 109 percent value as a starting point and move up or down in small increments for a period of time, making a mark on the seat post to keep track of your adjustments. Seat posts that have calibrated scales are available. Give each new height a chance—100 miles or more—and settle finally for the most comfortable seat height.

## ANKLING–FACT AND FANCY

Earlier we discussed in some detail the need to apply forces that have a good turning effect about the crank axis. We pointed out that the "stampers"—the riders who apply just vertical forces—are far from being the most efficient. Ways to improve the turning effect of pedal forces have centered around changes in the orientation of the pedal throughout the revolution of the cranks—a technique known to enthusiasts as "ankling." Unfortunately, some rather erroneous information on ankling has been perpetuated over the years. There have been very few experimental studies but a lot of speculation, some of it quite definitely misleading; particularly to the beginner who is anxious to acquire the correct technique. The contrast between what has been recommended and what experienced cyclists actually do is shown in Figure 7.8.

In the upper diagram, what has been recommended mainly involves pushing the pedal across the top dead center by dropping the heel and pulling across the bottom dead center by raising to heel. Try this once; in particular, see how much you can drop your heel at the top of the stroke. If your leg is anything like mine, you cannot drop it very far—certainly not far enough to really push in the manner indicated in the drawing.

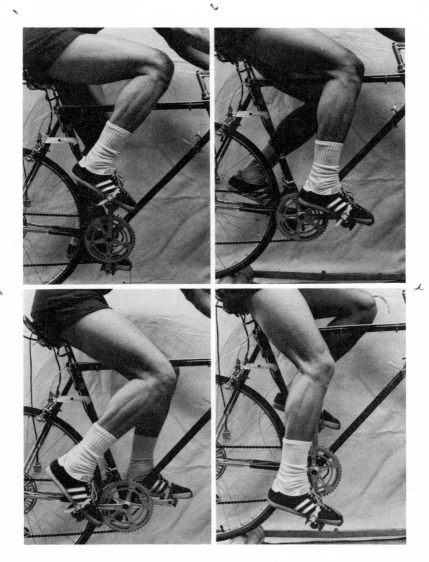

**FIGURE 7.7.** Four points in the pedalling cycle of a cyclist whose seat height is close to the physiologically determined optimal.

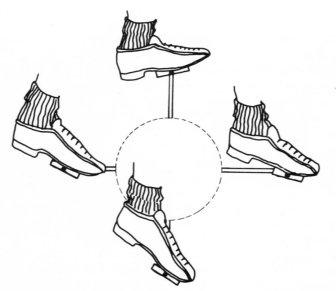

FIGURE 7.8. Above: The pattern of foot movement often recommended as the 'prefered' style of ankling.
Below: The actual pattern used, on average, by the racing cyclists tested at Penn State University.

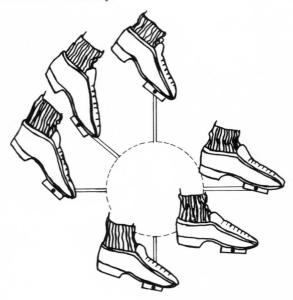

The lower part of Figure 7.8, what cyclists actually do, shows the mean patterns from 14 racing cyclists who we tested with the specially instrumented pedal shown in Figure 7.1. Notice what they do; we could characterize the style as toes-down pedalling, and this is very different indeed from the style in the upper diagram that was advocated by opinion and not experiment. The foot reaches its steepest inclination to the horizontal about 45 degrees before the top of the cycle. From that point onward, there is a gradual flattening through the first quadrant that ends halfway through the second quadrant when the foot is almost horizontal. When the work load is heavier, there is a slight tendency to put the heel down at this point, which corresponds roughly with the time of maximum force application. During recovery, the heel is gradually raised back to the high point at which this description began.

The opinion has been expressed by some that ankling styles in racing and touring are different but there is no evidence to confirm or deny this at the moment. It seems reasonable to recommend that you try out the toes-down pedalling style, which is shown in the lower part of figure 7.8 and forget the anatomically difficult "fancy" shown above. This technique should be practiced frequently, although it may feel very strange at first. The final result will allow you to change the orientation of the net force vector on the pedal as shown in Figure 7.2 and will result in a more efficient pedalling action.

A final word about a common pedalling fault in many beginners who do not have toe clips on their bikes. The usual position of the pedal in relation to the foot is shown in Figure 7.7 but some people slide the foot forward so that the pedal spindle is virtually underneath the ankle joint. There are two reasons why this is bad form; first, it does not allow the ankle to go through the movements shown in Figure 7.7, which are necessary to change the orientation of the force vector from being simply vertical. Second, electromyography of this kind of pedalling shows, as you might expect, that the gastrocnemius and soleus are virtually inactive, since the turning effects about the ankle are very small. This means that these powerful muscles are being ignored and prevented from contributing to the production of force. If you find yourself pedalling this way, then it might be a good idea to put toe clips onto your bike. They will keep your foot in the right position on the pedal during normal cycling and will be of help during those special efforts such as hill climbing when maximum output is required .

## WHAT FEELS GOOD MUST BE RIGHT

Pedalling speed, expressed in revolutions per minute, has been given much attention in the cycling literature. The speed at which the pedal crank is turned per minute can influence cycling efficiency, that is, the amount of work produced per liter of oxygen consumed. Both oxygen uptake and heart rate have been shown to be slightly higher while pedalling at 20 revolutions per minute as compared with 60 revolutions per minute for equivalent power outputs. Alterations in revolutions per minute between 50 and 80 revolutions per minute at equivalent power outputs do not substantially change the energy cost. However, energy cost at higher pedalling speeds, 100 to 120 revolutions per minute, is greater when compared to lower speeds at similar power outputs. In general, physiological responses indicate a metabolic similarity for cycling over a wide range of pedalling speeds, 40 to 80 revolutions per minute. Unfortunately, most of the data on pedalling rate have been derived using nonracing cyclists pedalling a stationary bicycle ergometer. The physical structure of the ergometer, that is, heavy flywheel, steel cranks, saddle to crank position, and so on, differs so much from the lightweight racing bicycle that conclusions drawn from such studies can hardly be applied to the cyclist on a racing bicycle. The "most efficient" pedalling rate for the nonracing cyclist pedalling a bicycle ergometer is always considerably lower than that preferred by the racing cyclist. However, trained racing cyclists who have been tested on bicycle ergometers have shown little difficulty handling loads at 90 to 120 revolutions per minute when attempting to achieve their highest power outputs and $VO_2$ maximum.

Empirical evidence suggests that most road-racing cyclists prefer crank speeds between 90 to 100 revolutions per minute. The trained cyclist selects the gear and revolution per minute that from experience "feels good" and appears to result in "optimum" performance. When the trained cyclist is made to vary plus or minus 20 revolutions per minute from the preferred crank revolution per minute, oxygen cost is increased by 10 to 15 percent. If asked to cycle in a large gear at a low revolution per minute, the cyclist complains of aching and tight thigh muscles. In fact, the tension developed in the quadriceps generally leads to premature fatigue. For example, muscles of the quadricep group fatigue before a maximal demand has been placed on the cardiopulmonary system. Thus, use of large gears at a slow crank speed is metabolically inefficient.

There exists an optimal relationship between the force developed and the pedalling frequency. The muscle force necessary to maintain equivalent power output increases as pedalling speed becomes slower but resistance greater. It has been demonstrated that oxygen cost at low-power development using high revolutions per minute against a small resistance is equivalent to that at much higher power development at slower revolutions per minute and against higher resistances. During prolonged cycling, high-power output is best gained through high pedalling rates.

The racing cyclist today is using larger gears than seen previously, yet maintaining high revolutions per minutes. There is evidence that peak efficiency may not be reached using even gears of 111 inches. This implies that perhaps the cyclist needs to continue to explore the use of gears larger than 111 inches, a practice significantly different from tradition. Remember that with the load held constant, the rate of oxygen consumption by the muscle cell is a  function of the frequency of contraction. Thus, oxygen uptake by the working muscle can be varied over the range of gear ratios by varying the revolutions per minute. Regardless of the gear ratio and revolution per minute selected, a smooth turning style is essential or torque output will fall significantly.

The question of blood flow to the working muscle during high pedalling rates has been raised. Some have suggested that high revolutions per minute may reduce blood flow to the working muscles. For the untrained cyclist, flow might be restricted, but research has indicated that blood flow to quadriceps muscles rises progressively with the increase in cycling intensity up to maximal effort. It is common knowledge that the racing cyclist can continue to pedal at 96 or greater revolutions per minute for at least two hours at work levels requiring an eightfold increase in oxygen uptake, 70 percent $VO_2$ maximum, without an appreciable rise in blood lactate. For the highly trained road-racing cyclist, muscular circulation does not appear to constitute a limiting factor for aerobic work. When, however, work is above 85 percent $VO_2$ maximum or supramaximal as during sprinting, blood flow may be restricted. Such restriction will then be a significant factor for limiting performance.

Coupled with increased revolutions per mimute is the greater need and use of stored muscle fuel. Therefore, the capacity to continue work at high intensity correlates well with the initial content of muscle fuel or glycogen. During prolonged, severe cycling effort, muscle fuel rather than crank speed will be the limiting factor.

## BIBLIOGRAPHY

Hamley E. J., and V. Thomas, "Physiological and Postural Factors in the Calibration of the Bicycle Ergometer." *J. Physiology, 191:* 55-57P (1967).

Shennum P.L., and H.A. deVries. "The effect of saddle height on oxygen consumption during bicycle ergometer work." *Medicine and Science in Sports, 8,* No. 2, 119-121 (1976).

Daly D.J., and P.R. Cavanagh. "Asymmetry in Bicycle Ergometer Pedalling." *Medicine and Science in Sports, 8,* No. 3, 204-208 (1976).

Gregor R.J., and P.R. Cavanagh. "Patterns of Force Application in Bicycle Riding." *Medicine and Science in Sports.* In press 1977.

# SECTION 8
# How Do I Train?

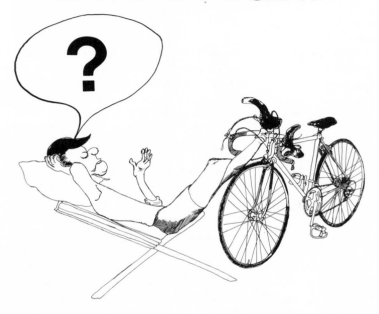

## GENERAL GUIDELINES

Achievement of high performance in the sport of cycling is possible only through systematic training that is structured according to known scientific laws and principles. Training for best results is based on three biological principles: (1) the overload principle; (2) the principle of specificity; and (3) the principle of reversibility of action.

The overload principle states that functional changes occur in the body only when the load is sufficient to cause considerable activization of energy exchange in the cells. The principle of specificity stipulates that functional and morphological changes during training occur only primarily in the organs, cells, and intracellular structures that receive the greatest part of the physical load. Finally, the principle of reverse action is based on the fact that physiological changes brought about by training are transitory in nature. Functional changes that follow cessation of work are restored to normal values. Both physiological and anatomic modifications of the body, acquired during the process of training, return to their initial state after cessation of regular training.

Training for cycling involves both instructional training and competitive training, during which the cyclist's objectives are: (1) to master technique and tactics; (2) to develop strength, endurance, and speed; (3) to develop emotional and volitional qualities; and (4) to gain experience. For some individuals, training through cycling is not enough but must be supplemented with general, physical-development exercises. These exercises serve for overall strengthening of the body, all-around physical development, and correction of defects in body build. Such exercises include weight training, running, and flexibility movements. As much as possible, these exercises should be similar in form and nature to the elements of cycling. Similar exercises allow the cyclist to selectively develop strength, speed, and joint mobility precisely as required for more effective cycling.

Various protocols are used in the training of the cyclist. Methods differ depending on the intensity of exercise, the duration of continuous work, and the interval between exercises. The "repetition overload" method is often adopted, which designates the repetition of exercise at given intensities and rest intervals. The protocol selected depends on the goal of the training. The training session usually consists of the warm-up, the main work periods, and the cool-down or concluding portion. Depending on the goal, the main work period consists of exercises for developing speed and technique, followed by exercises for strength and endurance development.

The physiological load or stress during the training session is usually determined by the pulse rate. First, there occurs a fairly rapid rise in pulse rate, with oscillations in the middle of the work interval (150 to 165 beats per minute), and then a gradual lowering of the rate during the final stages. Following the training session, the pulse rate should not exceed the normal rate by greater than 10 to 15 beats per minute.

The length of the workout session is usually an hour and a half but, depending on the selected type of training, it will vary; for example, 45 to 60 minutes for the sprinter and pursuitist in the competitive period, three to four hours for a road cyclist in the preparatory period. Another form of training is competition itself. Frequent participation in racing is an ideal way to enhance fortitude, pain tolerance, and the will to do one's best.

Workouts should be planned so that exercises for developing strength of the large muscle groups, improving flexibility, and acquiring specialized endurance take place at least three times per week. Exercises for training in specialized endurance with competitive or greater intensity should be performed only twice a week. Workouts for mastering technique with maximum effort, participation in competition, and active rest should be conducted one time a week.

In order to achieve noticeable changes in performance ability, the correct amount of rest is essential. Restorative processes begin immediately after work is stopped, and gradually increase. During a certain time of the rest period the restorative processes exceed the initial, prework level. This supercompensatory phase of the body's adaptation to an overload leads to an improved physiological state or a training effect.

At this time it is not possible to identify the exact onset of the supercompensatory phase nor its completion. However, certain restorative time processes have been identified. For example, approximately 30 minutes is required for the complete restoration of the creatin-phosphate reserves in the muscles after brief, intense work; restoration of intramuscular glycogen reserves, following intense cycling, takes about one and one-half to 2 hours. In addition, the supercompensatory phase that follows prolonged cycling is accompanied by considerable expenditure of carbohydrate and fat reserves in the body and usually takes about two to three days to be achieved after cycling.

Certainly it is not necessary to rest until there is total completion of the restorative processes in order to realize a training effect. In accordance with the overload principle, it is desirable to follow a protocol in which repetitive loads occur during the phase of incomplete restoration. Sufficient rest after this protocol will result in a much greater supercompensation than with a one-time work load.

Maintenance of the acquired trained state requires a certain amount of cycling. If there is a reduction in cycling below a certain critical amount the detraining phenomenon will begin. Likewise, there is a limit to the body's adaptive, accomodative capacity. When one attempts to exceed that limit, functional capacity begins to slip. The key to training then, is to plan a program that will allow the cyclist to peak at critical periods during the competitive season.

As the cyclist proceeds to train, those loads that produced the greatest physiological changes at the beginning of training will not do so later on. The beginning phase of functional adaptation takes place rather slowly, usually lasting four to six weeks. This general adaptative phase is followed by a specific adaptation to the given cycling training. This phase of training usually takes 6 to 12 weeks. Next comes the maintenance phase, which varies from three to six weeks. This phase is followed by the process of readaptation during which there may be some loss of functional capacity. At this time it appears that the body reaches a period of a low-adaptive reserve. This adaptive loss is a result of the functioning of the endocrine glands that serve to regulate the body's adaptive processes to stress.

During the readaptive phase the training effect is not lost. The lowering of physiological function is temporary. At this time the size of the training load should be varied to avoid an overtrained or de-training process. Soon, the individual will be ready to embark upon the next higher training load.

## AEROBIC AND ANAEROBIC TRAINING

The primary aim of training should be to improve cardiorespiratory adaptation to cycling. This means that the training program should emphasize the skills and energy systems that are used for cycling. As in most sports, two energy system, aerobic and anaerobic, are employed during cycling. These systems are discussed in Section 2. The term aerobic, you recall, implies that the rate of oxygen uptake is adequate to meet the oxygen needs of the working muscle cells as they utilize energy substrates of carbohydrates and fats. The aerobic system, remember, is predominatly used during long-term cycling, which is performed at a submaximal rate. A cyclist's aerobic power may be measured directly or be predicted by using maximal or submaximal testing procedures. An individual's maximum aerobic power or oxygen uptake ($\dot{V}O_2$ maximum) is determined by measuring the maximum amount of oxygen that he or she can utilize in a one-minute period while cycling at maximum intensity. The minute volume of oxygen utilized is then expressed in either absolute terms such as liters per minute (e.g., $\dot{V}O_2$ max = 3.8 1/min) or relative to body weight in kilograms (e.g., $\dot{V}O_2$ max = 64 ml/kg.min). Other measurements made during a $\dot{V}O_2$-maximum test include maximum-ventilation volume rate, blood lactate, and heart rate. Maximum-ventilation volume rate per minute ($\dot{V}E$) is a measure of the amount of air moved into and out of the cyclist's lungs per minute.

The term anaerobic, you may recall, relates to those metabolic processes that occur when oxygen is not at the disposal of the working muscle cells as they utilize energy substrates of carbohydrates in the form of glucose or glycogen. The anerobic system is predominatly used during short-term cycling, which is performed at supramaximal rates. The extent to which the anaerobic system is involved during exercise is indicated by blood-lactate levels.

Several factors including the intensity of cycling, the condition of the cyclist, riding experience (efficiency and technique), and duration of the ride determine whether and the extent to which the anaerobic or aerobic system is used. In addition, during work there is an interplay between anaerobic and aerobic metabolism. There is no abrupt shift from one system to another but a somewhat subtle transition. The two systems overlap as well as being influenced by diet and training. Figure 8-1 illustrates the transition process.

All training can be arranged on a time scale relative to the total time of the competitive event. Whether the objective is to cycle at maximum effort and intensity or a given percent of the maximum for the duration of the event, the metabolic energy sources necessary for the task can be estimated. Through the identification of the specific energy yielding system for a given cycling task, it is possible to train that system to provide the maximum energy necessary for the performance. If more than one of the energy yielding systems is to be conditioned, which is usually the case, the training time must be divided. However, regardless of the system(s) used, an overload is necessary for enhanced performance. In simple terms, an overload implies that the cyclist must train at an intensity beyond that which one is already capable.

A basic principle to follow when designing any training program is that the exercise employed should be designed to engage muscle groups in the movement patterns involved in cycling. Considering this principle, we should ask whether it is wise to engage in a running program. Running in this case is considered generalized training for endurance and therefore might be considered ill-advised and inefficient use of time. Training protocol should be designed according to the

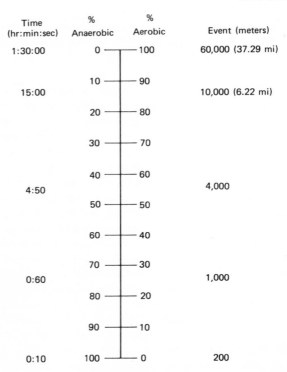

**FIGURE 8.1.** Aerobic and anaerobic energy system contribution in relation to distance and duration of the cycling event.

principle of specificity. The importance of selecting the appropriate exercises as they relate to the competitive situation includes such factors as intensity, pace, and duration, as well as tactics.

## TRAINING PROTOCOLS

Three primary approaches to training seem to dominate at this time. These are the LSD (long, slow-distance), steady-state, and interval approaches to training. For the most part the prevailing trend is adoption of the steady-state and interval program. For this reason the major portion of this discussion will center around steady-state and interval training.

Interval training is a system of conditioning in which the metabolic systems of the body are subjected to short but regularly repeated periods of work stress interspersed with designated relief periods. The overload principle may be applied to interval training through the manipulation of the following variables: (1) work duration; (2) relief interval time; (3) number of work intervals; (4) frequency of training per day; and (5) cycling distance.

There are an infinite number of interval-training combinations. The cyclist can select one or several training protocols, each of which produces a different training effect. Regardless of the protocol adopted, the intensity of the effort should, over time, be increased gradually as exercise tolerance permits, but always with adequate recovery. As one's physical condition improves, the dosage should be increased.

The importance of interval training or intermittent exercise in the development of both anaerobic and aerobic power of the body cannot be overemphasized. In interval training, the ratio between anaerobic and aerobic production of energy is about 1:3 for two-minute interval exercise and about 1:4 for four minute interval work. It appears quite clear that intermittent exercise improves both anoxidative and oxidative cycling capacity.

The advantage of intermittent or interval training over LSD and steady-state training is the number of times one can stress the body's metabolic systems. Also, cycling at a high intensity, but incorporating short spells of activity and rest, the work can be performed without or with only a comparatively slight increase in blood lactic-acid concentration. The short periods of work are energetically sustained by the breakdown of the energy-rich phosphate compounds of the muscle cell (ATP and creatine phosphate). With one-minute intervals, the glycolytic pathway plays only an unimportant role in energy metabolism. Conversely, two- to four- minute intervals result in high levels of lactate. This is due to either a marked breakdown of muscle glycogen or a high uptake of blood glucose by the muscle. Because the glucose output of the liver is not high enough to cover the energy requirements of the working muscles, the muscle glycogen must be the major energy source.

If the cycling portion of the interval lasts four minutes, 60 percent of the lactic-acid output is accounted for by the glucose extracted from the blood. The other 40 percent comes from muscle glycogen itself. This type of work strongly stimulates aerobic metabolism. During cycling periods of four minutes, 43 to 50 percent of the glycogen comes from the muscle while during two minutes of cycling, between 57 to 95 percent comes from the muscle. This rather short interval of two minutes stimulates anaerobic metabolism. When the cycling interval is 10 seconds or less, almost no lactic acid (alactic) is produced. Such sprint training stresses the anaerobic enzyme system. Stored oxygen plays an important role for the oxygen supply during such a short spell of hard cycling. This oxygen appears to be stored mainly in combination with myohemoglobin in the working muscles. At maximum effort, muscle contraction will last up to two minutes at a cost of about 16 kilocalories.

Another training program is the steady-state system. This type of training brings about several functional modifications. There is generally an increase in the heart's stroke volume and more complete extraction of oxygenated blood in the working muscles or a more economical use of oxygen in the blood. The intensity of effort in steady-state training is often at approximately 15 times the resting metabolic rate whereby all oxidation can be supplied by atmospheric oxygen. Steady-state training means constant effort for several minutes, generally 30 minutes or more, at a given level of intensity.

## TRAINING INTENSITY

The work load or intensity is generally expressed in percent of maximum oxygen uptake. Because the heart rate is generally related to oxygen uptake, it is possible to estimate the percent of maximum effort using the working heart rate. For example, to determine an effective training heart rate (THR) the formula developed by Karvonen may be used. The equation for computing the training heart rate is the following:

THR = MaxHR - RHR + (60% of difference between maximum and resting heart rate)
Example:
     MaxHR = 180
     RHR = - 60
     ──────────
            120
          ×0.60
     ──────────
          72.00

THR = 60 + 72 = 132 beats/min.

Although the Karvonen formula may be used as an accurate estimator of the training heart rate for the endurance cyclist, the environmental temperature or relative humidity must be considered. A high humidity or high environmental temperature would result in the estimated training heart rate being too low.

Various training studies suggest that the training threshold must exceed 140 heart beats per minute (close to 60% of the difference between the resting and maximal heart rate) if a significant training effect is to be elicited. For example, an exercise prescription for a cyclist with a resting heart rate of 50 and a maximal rate of 190 would be 0.60 (190 - 50) + 50 or 134 beats per minute. During steady-state work the training heart rate should be maintained for 30 minutes or more.

Maximal heart rate varies with age and sex of the individual. Table 8.1 presents this variance and may be used as a guide for estimating the training heart rate. A rough estimate of one's maximal heart rate may be determined by subtracting age in years from 220. Resting heart rate may be determined while sitting quietly in a chair after rising in the morning. Although maximum heart rate varies little with training, the resting heart rate typically decreases 10 to 20 beats after a month or more of training. A 10 to 20 beat drop, however, results in an insignificant change in the training heart rate.

To determine the working heart rate, the cyclist should take her or his pulse rate during the first 10 seconds of recovery. The obtained figure is then multiplied by six in order to obtain the number of beats per minute. Take 2 percent of the minute figure and add it to itself. This added 2 percent will serve to decrease the error of the estimate. A more exact but difficult procedure for some is to determine the working pulse while cycling. Whichever method is selected, the pulse may be determined by using the palpitation technique of counting the carotid or apical pulse. A descending tendency in the heart rate measured at postexercise after cycling of equal intensity indicates improved economy of the cardiopulmonary system.

## STRESSING A SYSTEM

During steady-state training any sudden increase in speed or load, for example, climbing, jams, and so on, will produce a quantity of lactate in the quadriceps muscles of the thigh. The lactate increase is due to the inability of the oxygen delivery system to respond immediately to any increased work demand. During this initial time lag, working muscles draw on stored oxygen until more oxygen can be supplied (oxygen-deficit period). The greater the increase in cycling intensity, the more it is necessary for anaerobic glycolysis to produce energy (ATP); and therefore the greater will be the production of lactic acid. With high lactic-acid levels, muscular contraction is inhibited and depletion of glycogen stores means the muscle has run out of fuel.

It takes a minimum of two minutes for the energy supplying system to adjust to a new level of cycling intensity. If a new level of cycling intensity is beyond the aerobic capcity of the cyclist, the legs begin to hurt and breathing becomes rapped. These are signs of lactate acidosis caused by a lack of oxygen and lactate generation. The cyclist will soon reach a point when it is impossible to continue at the new pace and he or she must slow down to pay back the oxygen debt incurred.

**TABLE 8.1.** Maximum mean heart rate for age and training heart rate at 60 percent.

| AGE (yr) | MAX HR RANGE (bpm) | MEAN | THR*a |
|---|---|---|---|
| 10 | 190-200 | 205 | 147 |
| 15 | 185-218 | 203 | 145 |
| 20-29 | 173-213 | 193 | 139 |
| 30-39 | 165-205 | 185 | 135 |
| 40-49 | 156-196 | 176 | 129 |
| 50-59 | 148-188 | 168 | 124 |
| 60-69 | 141-181 | 161 | 120 |
| 70-79 | 133-153 | 153 | 115 |
| 80-89 | 125-145 | 145 | 111 |

a*THR = training heart rate at 60% maximum of mean heart rate using resting heart rate of 60 beats per minute.

The lactic acid produced during the oxygen-deficit period must now be disposed of, which requires the use of additional energy (ATP). Most of the lactic acid diffuses from the muscle cells into the blood where it is carried to the liver, heart, and muscles. Eighty to ninety percent of the lactic acid is turned back into glycogen in the liver to be later used for energy production. The remaining 10 to 20 percent is used to provide the energy to reconvert lactic acid to glycogen.

It is obvious that the energy liberated by the production of lactate from glycogen does not equal the energy required to recycle lactate into glycogen. Because of this fact, a substantial amount of "extra energy" could be used during long races for purposes other than muscle contraction. It is recommended, therefore, that during long races or rides a steady pace be maintained as much as possible. In addition, the cyclist should develop an aerobic system that will cycle at a high intensity without relying on anaerobic energy.

A review of racing events indicates that pursuiters gain approximately 60 percent of their total energy from lactate production. The kilometer riders and time trialist obtain about 90 percent of their energy anaerobically, while the road racers gain up to 100 percent of their energy aerobically. The kilometer rider and time trialist might give less importance to aerobic training but cannot completely ignore such training. Aerobic processes, it will be recalled, are essential for recovery. Although road racing is primarily aerobic, the jumps, breakaways, and end sprints require anaerobic power, which makes it essential for successful road racing. Generally, the racing cyclist should have the ability to produce energy aerobically as well as anaerobically and to tolerate high lactate concentrations.

Evidence has been accumulated substantiating the conclusion that regular training of a progressive intensity is an effective training program. An infinite variety of training protocols for the pursuit, time trial, and road cyclist have been published, but as yet none have been scientifically tested. Table 8.2 presents example training protocols designed to stress a given energy producing system. Remember that the length of the individual work period is most critical, while the length of the rest pauses and the work output are of secondary importance.

The ability to "jam" or effectively execute a sudden sprint is essential during a race. When there is an attempted breakaway or during a turn, the cyclist must suddenly increase the revolutions per minute approximately 20 to 30 percent. Special training is necessary for achieving effective sudden acceleration. Examples of acceleration training are the following: (1) accelerate from 25 to 55 kilometers per hour; rest five minutes between four work intervals; and (2) accelerate from 35 to 55 kilometers and maintain 55 kilometers for approximately 10 seconds, repeating the work interval five times.

**TABLE 8.2.** Anaerobic and aerobic training protocols

| SYSTEM STRESSED | WORK | REST | REPETITIONS |
|---|---|---|---|
| Anaerobic-Enzyme alactic | 10 sec | 20 sec | 25-40 |
| Anaerobic-Lactic acid | 30 sec | 30 sec | 20-30 |
| | 45 sec | 30 sec | 20-30 |
| | 60 sec | 60 sec | 15-20 |
| | 60 sec | 15 sec | 15-20 |
| Aerobic | 3 min | 3 min | 10-15 |
| | 5 min | 5 min | 10-15 |
| | 10 min | 5 min | 6-8 |
| | 15 min | 5 min | 4-6 |

Steady-state training should be incorporated into an interval program at least twice a week. Such training might take the form of time trials. The course selected should be a 30- to 90-minute ride while a 30-minute hilly course should be sufficient. An example of a two-week, preracing-season training program is the following:

Two-Week, Pre Racing-Season Training Program
Sunday—120 to 160 kilometers
Monday—Weight training; aerobic intervals
Tuesday—Time trial—hilly course
Wednesday—Weight training; anaerobic intervals
Thursday—Anaerobic intervals
Friday—Weight training; aerobic intervals
Saturday—Rest or light riding
Sunday—120 to 160 kilometers (some hills)
Monday—Weight training; anaerobic intervals
Tuesday—Acceleration training
Wednesday—Weight training; anaerobic intervals
Thursday—Time trialing—flat course
Friday—Weight training—aerobic intervals
Saturday—Rest or light riding

Riding should be at 80 to 100 revolutions per minute while incorporating the use of a 70-inch gear for low-gear intervals. Training is made more enjoyable with a partner of comparable ability. Trade-off riding during both interval and steady-state training will allow each rider to present to the other an additional challenge of the pain threshhold. The frequency of training might begin three days per week but, as conditioning takes place, a five-day training schedule with one racing day is essential for maximum results.

The advantage of intermittent training is the number of times the cyclist can stress a given system. By cycling at high intensity but incorporating short periods of work and recovery, the work can be performed with or without only a comparatively slight increase in blood lactic-acid concentration. As the trained state develops, the cyclist can withstand longer total work periods without complete exhaustion.

Of course the substrate used during training will depend on the intensity and duration of the work intervals as well as on total training-session time. Periods of two to four minutes result either in a marked breakdown of muscle glycogen or a high uptake of blood glucose by the muscle cells. Because the glucose output of the liver is not high enough to cover the energy requirement of the working muscles, the muscle glycogen must be the major energy source.

In addition to glycogen use, plasma-free fatty acid (FFA) levels of the arterial blood fall at the beginning of cycling. This fall is followed by a rise in plasma FFA. Such changes reflect first an increased uptake and utilization of FFA in the skeletal muscle and other organs, and second, the mobilization of FFA from adipose tissue. The mobilization of FFA during intermittent cycling will increase with increasing duration of cycling intervals. On the other hand, continuous cycling at high intensity (e.g., 75% $\dot{V}O_2$ max) is accompanied by a reduction of the utilization of fat as an energy source by the muscle, in favor of carbohydrates. As conditioning progresses, the trained cyclist becomes capable of work at 85-percent $\dot{V}O_2$ maximum without calling upon the glycolytic system.

## MUSCLE FIBER TYPES

There are more than 400 voluntary (skeletal, striped or striated) muscles in the human body that constitute about 40 percent of the total body weight. Each skeletal muscle is composed of many thousands of individual contractile fibers. Not all of the muscle fibers of humans or animals have the same metabolic or functional capabilities. Although all fibers can function under both aerobic (with oxygen) and anaerobic (without oxygen) conditions, some fibers possess a unique biochemical structure enabling them to function better aerobically, whereas others are equipped to work anaerobically.

Recent application of histochemical and biochemical technique to human muscle has resulted in the identification of fast-twitch and slow-twitch fibers based on their contractile characteristics. The broad, glycogen-loaded, fast-twitch fibers function anaerobically, while the narrow, mitochondrial-rich, slow-twitch fibers function aerobically. When stimulated, the slow-twitch fiber can contract repeatedly without much fatigue. It contains a high content of myoglobin (an oxygen storing protein) and thus has a high aerobic or oxygen using capacity. This capacity is the muscle cell's ability to produce energy (ATP) at a steady rate for long durations when sufficient oxygen is available to it. The ability to accomplish such energy production is due to its large number of mitochondria, which are subcellular particles known as the "powerhouse" of the cell because of their energy producing activities.

The fast-twitch fiber, low in both myoglobin and mitochondrial concentration, fatigues easily; however, it functions at very high intensity during short work periods. This fiber type is preferentially recruited for performing short, high-intensity work such as sprinting. On the contrary, the slow-twitch fibers are preferentially recruited during long-term, endurance work.

Relatively, the average human has 40 to 50 percent slow-twitch fibers and 50 to 60 percent fast-twitch fibers. Sprint—and endurance—trained athletes are characterized by muscles with distinct fiber compositions and enzyme activities. Endurance athletes possess a majority of slow-twitch muscle fibers. For example, world-class marathoners have been found to have over 80 percent slow-twitch fibers and a world-class road cyclist indicated 73 percent slow-twitch fibers. In contract, those who excell in sprinting ability possess a larger percentage of fast-twitch fibers.

The cyclist's potential for sprinting or high-intensity, steady-state riding may be estimated by employing the muscle biopsy-technique. This is a simple procedure where, after local anesthesia, a needle-biopsy muscle sample is taken. After staining, a cross section of the muscle cell is microscopically viewed. Those cells staining dark are fast-twitch fibers while those remaining light are slow-twitch fibers. Fiber type dominance can then be easily identified. A predominance of fast-twitch fibers will give the cyclist an edge for anaerobic or sprint work. If the biopsy study indicates predominately slow-twitch fibers the cyclist's edge is for aerobic or long-term work.

Once fiber typing is completed, the training protocol may be structured to enhance either or both aerobic and anaerobic capacities of the muscle, depending on the cycling event. Either the inherent qualities of the muscle may be trained or one may wish to improve weaknesses.

Different training regimens enhance the anaerobic or aerobic capacity of a given fiber type. High-intensity, short-interval training increases the glycolytic capacity, anaerobic power, and size of the fast-twitch fibers. Aerobic training involving longer intervals or steady-state cycling stresses the slow-twitch fibers, thereby improving endurance or oxidative capacity of the slow-twitch muscle cells. It appears that high-intensity anaerobic training enhances the metabolic enzyme activity (phosphorylase) essential for anaerobic work or sprinting. On the other hand, long-term or endurance training appears to increase the number of fibers with high oxidative capacities. The question often raised is whether certain types of training will alter the percentage distribution of a specific fiber type. It appears that fiber composition, for example, contractile characteristics, is established early in life. Training only alters the metabolic qualities of the fibers.

There is a strong relationship between the oxidative or aerobic enzyme, succinate dehydrogenase (SDH), activity and oxygen uptake capacity. This fact suggests that endurance training enhances both the oxidative potential of skeletal muscle and physical working capacity.

Not every cyclist has the opportunity to have a muscle biopsy performed. However, it has been established that successful sprint- and endurance-trained athletes are distinguished by possessing distinct fiber types. With this knowledge and personal racing experience, the cyclist has a fair perception of strengths and weaknesses. If one is always dropped on the sprints and has trouble holding a position on a breakaway, it is obvious that the weakness lies in anaerobic capacity. To the contrary, if the cyclist has difficulty holding a position during a road race, the weakness lies in aerobic power. When the weakness is realized, the cyclist need only select a specific training regime.

Finally, each must be aware that regardless of the muscle-cell fiber type, oxygen-transport or tissue-oxygen utilization are significant factors limiting oxygen consumption during maximal cycling. In the end it is often training plus the cyclist's genetic endurance that determine success. The successful road racer needs aerobic power to conquer the long distance and anaerobic power to sprint at the finish.

## ASSESSING AEROBIC POWER

Prior to beginning a training program, the approximation of each cyclist's initial aerobic capacity should be known. This may be accomplished through the use of a laboratory, oxygen uptake capacity test or by using one of the predictive methods. Test results serve to establish beginning levels of training intensity and, if repeated at intervals, the data will provide help in determining the effectiveness of the training program. In addition, test data will allow for training protocols to be tailored to the individual cyclist.

Most colleges and universities as well as some YMCAs have the necessary laboratory equipment to perform oxygen-uptake tests. Generally, a medical clearance from a personal physician is necessary before the test can be administered. If laboratory facilities are not available, a predictive oxygen-uptake test may be substituted. The 12-minute-run test as described by Kenneth Cooper, author of *The New Aerobics*, is an effective test for estimating oxygen-uptake capacity. Another method for predicting aerobic power is bench stepping, from which the pulse rate is plotted on a nomogram. The testing procedure and scoring method is described by Mathews and Fox in their text, *The Physiological Basis of Physical Education and Athletics.* Use of the Åstrand-Ryhming nomogram will produce a standard deviation from the direct measured maximal oxygen uptake of $\pm$ 15 percent.

Endurance or aerobic power is essential for all cyclists whether they are engaged in long-term cycling or sprint cycling. Therefore endurance training is essential for all cyclists. Aerobic training will produce a higher cardiac functional reserve in order to meet those high-stress moments during cycling. In addition, the cyclist will have the potential to work at a higher metabolic level without encountering the problems brought about by metabolic waste products, that is, lactic acid. The greater the aerobic power the higher the rate of energy expenditure the cyclist can maintain before encountering fatigue.

## BIBLIOGRAPHY

Åstrand, P.O., and K. Rodahl. *Textbook of Work Physiology*. McGraw-Hill, New York, 1970.

Barnard, R. J., V. R. Edgerton, and J. B. Peter. "Effect of Exercise on Skeletal Muscle, I. Biochemical and Histochemical Properties. "*J. Appl. Physiol., 28*: 762-766 (1970).

Burke, E., and B. Fink. "What Muscle Fiber Type Are You?". *Bike World, 4:* 48-50 (1975).

Cooper, K. H. *The New Aerobics*. Bantam Books, New York. 1970.

Costill, D. L., J. Daniels, W. Evans, W. Fink, G. Krahenbuhl, and B. Saltin. "Skeletal Muscle Enzymes and Fiber Composition in Male and Female Track Athletes." *J. Appl. Physiol., 40:* 149-154 (1976).

Costill, D. L., P. D. Gollnick, E. D. Jansson, B. Saltin, and E. M. Stein. "Glycogen Depletion Patterns in Human Muscle Fibers During Distance Running." *Acta Physiol. Scand., 89:* 374-383 (1973).

Davis, J. A., and V. A. Convertino. "A Comparison of Heart Rate Methods for Predicting Endurance Training Intensity." *Med. Sci. Sports, 7:* 295-298 (1975).

Eriksson, B. O., P. D. Gollnick, and B. Saltin. "Muscle Metabolism and Enzyme Activities After Training in Boys 11-13 Years Old." *Acta Physiol. Scand., 87:* 231-239 (1972).

Engel, W. K., and M. H. Brooke. "Muscle Biopsy as a Clinical Diagnosis Aid." In: *Neurological Diagnostic Techniques,* edited by W. S. Field. Thomas, Springfield, Ill. 1966, pp. 90-146.

Faria, I. E. "Cardiovascular Response to Exercise as Influenced by Training of Various Intensities." *Res. Quart., 41:* 44-50 (1970).

Gollnick, P. D., R. B. Armstrong, C. W. Saubert, IV, K. Piehl, and B. Saltin. "Enzyme Activitiy and Fiber Composition in Skeletal Muscle of Untrained and Trained Men." *J. Appl. Physiol., 33:* 312-319 (1972).

Karvonen, M. J., E. Kentala, and O. Mustala. "The Effects of Training on Heart Rate, A Longitudinal Study." *Ann. Med. Exper. Fenn., 35:* 307-315 (1957).

Mathews, D. K., and E. L. Fox. *The Physiological Basis of Physical Education and Athletics*. W. B. Saunders, Philadelphia, 1976. pp. 507-509.

Morgan, T. E., L. A. Cobb, F. A. Short, R. Ross, and D. R. Gunn. "Effects of Long-Term Exercise on Human Muscle Mitochondria." In: *Muscle Metabolism During Exercise,* edited by B. Pernow and B. Saltin. Plenum, N. Y., 1971. pp. 87-95.

Saltin, B. "Metabolic Fundamentals in Exercise." *Med. Sci. Sports, 5:* 137-146 (1973).

Sharkey, B. J., and J. P. Hollenman. "Cardiorespiratory Adaptations to Training at Specific Intensities." *Res. Quart., 38:* 698-704 (1967).

Shephard, R. J. "Intensity, Duration, and Frequency of Exercise as Determinants of the Response to a Training Regimen." *Int. Z. Angew. Physiol., 26:* 272-278 (1968).

Volkov, N. "The Logic of Sports Training." *Track and Field, 10:* 22-23 (1974).

# SECTION 9
# The Cyclist's Diet

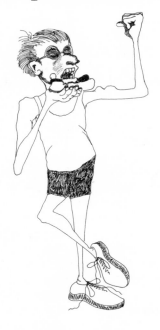

The bicycle is a remarkably efficient machine. It affords an opportunity for an individual to move her or his body weight in an energy conserving manner. Researchers have compiled data on the energy consumed in moving a certain distance as a function of body weight. From these data it became quite clear that an individual on a bicycle reduces walking energy consumption to about a fifth (0.15 calories per gram per kilometer) of normal. This energy expenditure for movement places humans on a bicycle first among moving creatures and machines.

With the above discussion in mind, let us now examine various foods and their use as energy producing substrates. All energy from food is convertible to heat; therefore, it is usually measured as heat. A unit of heat energy is known as a calorie, which is the heat required to raise the temperature of 1 gram of water one centigrade degree. The term kilocalorie (kcal), which is 1000 small calories, is used to express the amount of energy to be found in foods. For example, a banana contains about 85 kilocalories.

The energy required during a two-hour cycling race is approximately 3000 kilocalories. This value would of course vary with the type of terrain, environmental conditions, and cycling speed. Three-thousand kilocalories is significantly more energy than the average individual requires during a normal 24-hour period. The food that may be eaten during a race is small, if any. Therefore, the cyclist must rely on energy stores to supply the fuel the body requires to sustain high-intensity, long-duration muscle work.

The active muscle cells make use of intracellular storage depots in the form of glycogen or lipids. The vascular system provides additional fuel and oxygen. Remember that fuel and oxygen are utilized by the cells in metabolic reactions that generate adenosine triphosphate (ATP).

In the absence of a fuel substrate, the various metabolic pathways cannot provide the necessary energy for the work of cycling. Carbohydrate, in the form of glucose or glycogen, and fat, in the form of triglycerides (fatty acid plus glycerol), serve as fuel for energy production. Triglycerides are found stored mainly in adipose tissue and the liver. The extent to which fat and carbohydrate participate in the energy-production process depends upon several factors, such as the severity and duration of cycling in relation to the cyclist's maximal aerobic power and diet. For example, as the duration of cycling increases up to several hours, fat metabolism contributes up to 70 percent of the energy needed. If the cyclist increases the work intensity to the point of anaerobic involvement, carbohydrate will be the primary energy source. In this instance, the blood lactate produced from anaerobic-metabolic processes has the tendency to inhibit fat mobilization as does high blood-sugar levels.

Duration, intensity, and frequency of riding are factors to be considered when discussing the cyclist's diet. In general, a diet high (90%) in carbohydrate will permit the cyclist to work longer than a diet of high-fat content. Since it appears that the blood-sugar level is associated with work duration for the central nervous system, optimum blood-sugar levels are required for it to function properly. Stored muscle glycogen can serve to maintain the blood-sugar level to meet the needs of the central nervous system. It has been demonstrated that increased muscle-glycogen stores serve to increase the endurance capactiy or aerobic power of the cyclist. Research indicates that the muscle is capable of glycogen overcompensation if first depleted of its glycogen stores.

Muscle-glycogen stores may be depleted by engaging in prolonged heavy cycling for a three-day period while maintaining a low-carbo-hydrate diet. Overcompensation is accomplished by reducing the cycling activity for two to three days following depletion and main-taining a high-carbohydrate diet. For glycogen loading, complex carbo-hydrate rather than processed sugar foods are recommended. Complex carbohydrate foods include potatoes, rice, corn, whole wheat foods, and fruit. Through following the procedure described, it is possible to almost triple the muscle-glycogen stores. Therefore, the riding time in a 40-mile road race could be improved significantly. It appears that the glycogen—loading process is maximally effective not more than once a month.

Prior to engaging in the practice of carbohydrate or glycogen loading, the consequences should be clearly understood. With each gram of glycogen stored, there are 2.7 grams of water. The deposition of nearly three times as much water as glycogen adds body weight, which could in some instances be deleterious to the cyclist's performance. Glycogen and water can be deposited in the muscle to such an extent that a sensa-tion of heaviness and stiffness is produced. In a few instances, glycogen loading has resulted in the development of leg cramps or severe fatigue to the point of forcing the athlete to stop exercising. The cause of this fatigue has been attributed to muscle breakdown and an increase in myoglobin in the circulating blood to the point of clogging the kidneys and causing renal shutdown. It has been said that this phenomenon results from the effects of the first three days of low-carbohydrate intake accompanied by continued training. Recently, glycogen loading has been shown to alter the supply and utilization of fat-derived fuels during exercise. It decreases glycerol and plasma, free fatty acid con-centrations and increases ketone body concentration and insulin, and growth hormone levels. When practiced, the loading process is maxi-mally effective not more than once a month. Therefore, although the procedure is an effective, work-enhancing process, it exerts metabolic effects that could lead to reduced performance. It is recommended that if glycogen loading is going to be practiced, it should be experienced once or twice before engaging in the process for actual comptetition. This trial period will allow one to observe any unusual or negative side effects. In most instances the process should lead to positive results.

The longer the stores of glycogen last, the longer the duration cycling may be maintained. At what point during cycling the body calls upon muscle glycogen depends on the trained state of the cyclist and the intensity of cycling. The greater the aerobic power of the cyclist, the closer he or she can work to the maximum oxygen-uptake capacity without elevating the blood-lactate level. For example, the untrained cyclist begins to accumulate blood lactate at work loads of 40 to 50 percent of the individual maximal aerobic power whereas the trained cyclist may work at intensities as high as 65 to 70 percent maximum aerobic power without a significant elevation of blood lactate. For the cyclist it means that endurance training, in addition to increasing maximum oxygen-uptake capacity, results in the cyclist's ability to perform longer at a higher intensity. If at high cycling intensity less lactic acid is produced, fat mobilization will be inhibited to a lesser extent. Therefore, the glycogen stores will be depleted at a reduced rate while the fuel for muscle work is being derived from the fat stores. Thus, a glycogen-conserving process is in effect.

To sustain energy output of long duration — one hour or more — both intramuscular and extramuscular substrate utilization is necessary. The primary energy substrates used during cycling are fat and carbohydrate (CHO). Free fatty acids (FFA) are the major substrate used to support energy expenditure during long-duration cycling. Adipose tissue, by rapid release of free fatty acids, provides fuel for muscle contraction. The extent to which free fatty acids or fat and carbohydrate are mobilized and utilized is influenced by the metabolic rate induced by the stress of cycling. With prolonged cycling, there is an increase in free fatty acid mobilization resulting in a rise in plasma free fatty acid concentration. This rise progresses as long as the effort is of moderate intensity, less than 70 percent $\dot{V}O_2$ maximum.

Glucose too is important to muscle work. The development of hypoglycemia, low blood sugar, during a ride can seriously limit cycling endurance. Plasma glucose and central nervous system (CNS) glucose are maintained by means of glycogenolysis and release of liver glucose. Muscle glycogen is an energy source for muscle as well as a substrate for the central nervous system in prolonged cycling. Depletion of muscle glycogen leads to exhaustion and termination of work. The endurance limit, therefore, of the cyclist depends on the intensity of the effort and the initial glycogen contents of the liver and muscle. The well-conditioned cyclist, however, is better able to mobilize and oxidize free fatty acids for energy production. This ability serves to conserve liver and muscle glycogen. It should be pointed out that lactic acid interferes with free fatty acid mobilization from adipose tissue during work. This means that the intensity of effort, the percent $\dot{V}O_2$ maximum, must be judged carefully in order not to involve the anaerobic energy producing system to any great extent if one intends to conserve glycogen.

The roll of fat and carbohydrate metabolism during prolonged exhaustive work has been examined by various researchers. Attempts have been made to assess the degree of glycogen (carbohydrate) and free-fatty-acid (FFA, fat) utilization during various work intensities and durations. For example, when cycling at 75 percent maximal oxygen uptake ($\dot{V}O_2$ max), glycogen content in the vastus lateralis of the quadriceps-femoris muscle (primary cycling muscle of the upper leg) decreases approximately 30 percent per 100 grams of tissue within the first 15 minutes. During one hour of cycling at 80 percent $\dot{V}O_2$ maximum, glycogen decrease is as high as 64 percent per 100 grams of tissue.

During long-duration cycling at 75 to 80 percent of the cyclists $\dot{V}O_2$ maximum, the body shifts during the latter portion of the ride from glycogen utilization to the mobilization and utilization of fat. In contrast, with the beginning of cycling, approximately 90 percent of the oxygen consumed is used to metabolize carbohydrates. By the end of a long race, carbohydrate involvement in the energy producing system declines to approximately 67 percent. During relatively high-intensity (60 to 70% $\dot{V}O_2$ max), steady-state cycling for long durations (three to four hours), there occurs a shift from carbohydrate to lipid mobiliation and utilization for energy production.

It should be pointed out that there is a difference between glycogen utilization for running and cycling. During cycling a smaller muscle mass is involved than for running. Consequently, if the cyclist wishes to perform at the same percent of $\dot{V}O_2$ maximum as a runner, there will be greater stress placed on the quadriceps. The result is a greater degree of glycogen utilization for cycling than running. When compared to running, the cyclist is not able to work as long at about 80 percent of $\dot{V}O_2$ maximum without experiencing total muscle-glycogen depletion.

If the initial glycogen content of the working muscle is closely cor-rellated to cycling time to exhaustion and if glycogen loading can im-prove the cyclist's capacity for prolonged hard work, what then is the effect of diet during cycling of long duration?

Carbohydrate ingestion during hard cycling for several hours bene-fits performance. Glucose taken during cycling serves to maintain a satisfactory blood-sugar level, thereby reducing the work of the liver. Raised blood-glucose level during work appears to benefit the cen-tral nervous system. When glycogen stores are significantly reduced during prolonged heavy cycling, prolonged work can still be performed on submaximal levels provided that the supply of free fatty acids is adequate.

The cyclist must realize that at work rates above 65 to 70 percent of one's maximal oxygen uptake, there is a very high rate of glycogen breakdown, Also, even at heavy work loads, free fatty acids may ac-acount for as much as 30 percent of energy producing metabolic processes.

High-protein intake has been practiced by those claiming a need for added muscle strength. Excessive protein intake, however, has not proven beneficial. On the other hand, high-protein diets have produced mild to severe chronic nephritis and increased blood-urea concentra-tion. Since the metabolic cost of obtaining calories from protein ex-ceeds the cost from carbohydrate and fat, excessive protein consump-tion wastes body energy. The athlete needs no more than 0.8 grams of protein per kilogram of body weight during a 24-hour period as suggest-ed by the Food and Nutrition Board of the National Academy of Sciences. The ordinary diet provides this suggested intake level. From the evidence available there appears to be no place in the training of athletes for a high-protein diet or protein or amino-acid supplements.

## VITAMIN NEEDS

Natural vitamins are organic food substances found only in living things, that is, plants and animals. Vitamins are generally required in the diet in rather small amounts for normal growth, maintenance, and reproduction. They are not used for structural or energy require-ments nor as raw material for synthesizing processes. Although they have no caloric or energy value they are important to the body as con-situents of enzymes that function as catalysts in many metabolic reactions. In this role, vitamins assist with the regulation of metabolism, help convert fat and carbohydrates into energy, and assist in bone and tissue growth.

Daily, dietary vitamin requirements may not be absolute but are governed by the metabolic demands of the individual. Some vitamins are stored in the body in readiness for periods of inadequate intake. For example, the liver serves as a storage organ for vitamins A, D, $B_{12}$ and folic acid, while white blood cells store vitamin C and $B_2$.

Increased body requirements for vitamins have been recognized during periods of pregnancy lactation, growth, aging, and convalescence. The need for additional vitamin intake during periods of intense physical training and competition remains controversial. With the exceptions of vitamins A and D, excessive vitamin intake has thus far proved to be harmless.

Individual requirements for vitamins vary according to age, sex, body size, genetic makeup, and amount of physical activiy. It appears that with increased metabolic demands, there is a need for increased vitamin intake. For instance, the B-complex vitamins are active in providing the body with energy. Their involvement is principally associated with the conversion of carbohydrates into glucose and in the metabolism of fats and protein.

The B vitamin, except for $B_{17}$, are natural constituents of brewer's yeast, liver, or whole-grain cereals. Of these, brewer's yeast is the richest natural source of the B-complex group. The B-complex vitamins are water-soluble; therefore, they must be continually replaced. For purposes of identification the B-complex vitamins are $B_1$ (thiamine), $B_2$ (riboflavin), $B_3$ (niacin), $B_6$ (pyridoxine), $B_{12}$ (cyanocobalamin), $B_{13}$ (orotic acid), $B_{15}$ (pangamic acid), $B_{17}$ (laetrile), biotin, choline, folic acid, inositol, and PABA (para-aminobenzoic acid).

If the decision is made that the cyclist needs additional B-complex vitamins, it is important that all the B vitamins be taken together. Because of their interaction in functon, too much of any one of the B-complex group may cause another's deficiency. Vitamin balance is essential.

In endurance sports such as cycling, vitamin A, the B-complex group, C, E, and P appear to be the most important. Because of its role in the functional maintenance of the adrenal cortex, which plays a central role during stress, vitamin A intake for the athlete is recommended at 3 to 4 milligrams per day. Vitamin A sources are fish-liver oil, cream, butter, carrots, beet greens, spinach, and broccoli.

The vitamin B-complex group appear to be especially sensitive to endurance performance. Thiamine ($B_1$) is needed during periods of increased caloric use. The suggested daily requirement for the endurance athlete is 6 to 8 milligrams according to calories burned. It appears that thiamine is exhausted with large increases in metabolism. Good thiamine sources are lean pork, dry beans and peas, organ meats, some nuts, whole wheat and enriched cereals and bread.

Vitamin $B_2$ — riboflavin — combines with protein to form the important coenzymes, flavoproteins. The flavoproteins function in the respiration of tissue and act closely with the enzymes containing niacin. During periods of high performance, the daily requirement of 2 to 4 milligrams is indicated. Good riboflavin sources are milk, liver, heart, kidney, cheese, eggs, leafy green vegetables, and whole grain cereals.

For the building and reduction of carbohydrates and fats, niacin ($B_3$) is indispensible. Nicotinic acid or niacin in excess, however, inhibits the uptake of fatty acids by cardiac muscles during exercise. Since fatty acids are important fuels of the heart, vitamin supplements containing niacin are contraindicated before strenous cycling. The recommended daily intake is 40 milligrams for endurance work. Some sources of $B_3$ are lean meat and poultry, peanuts (excellent), beans, peas, whole grains and enriched cereal.

For the endurance cyclist, ascorbic acid (vitamin C) may amount to 500 milligrams daily. It appears that vitamin C, found in fruit juices, assists in ridding the body of lactic acid. Like C, vitamin E (tocopherols), has been somewhat controversial because of the claim that it influences circulation and capillarization, both of which improve the utilization of oxygen. The recommended vitamin E intake is perhaps 10 to 30 milligrams per day. Excellent sources of vitamin E are wheat germ and wheat germ oil, and whole grains.

The P-complex vitamins—rutin, citrin, and hesperidin—are essentially vitamin C stablizers. These bioflavonoids appear in fruits and vegetables as vitamin C companions. The bioflavonoids are, for example, found in lemons, grapes, plums, grapefruit, apricots, blackberries, and cherries. It appears quite clear that vitamin P serves to increase the strength of the capillaries and regulates their permeability.

The important point to be made is that vitamin supplementation per se will not increase endurance capacity. The issue is establishing a vitamin balance that will meet metabolic demands. It is basically agreed that an endurance cyclist who has a balanced diet cannot gain a specific advantage by taking food supplements; however, to perform at maximum potential, maximum dietary maintenance is essential. If, because of increased metabolic work, the body is left with dietary needs above normal daily expectations, nutritional supplementation may be recommended.

Excess water-soluble vitamins, that is, niacin, thiamine, riboflavin, and ascorbic acid, are excreted in the urine. The fat-soluble vitamins (A, D, E, K) are stored in the liver. Significant increases of the fat-soluble vitamins A and D have produced toxic effects. Several of the vitamins, including both fat- and water-soluble ones (C, E, K, and B-complex) are intimately involved in metabolic energy producing reactions. It seems logical then that high metabolic activity would require more than the average recommended vitamin intake. It is very likely that additional vitamin-cofactor linkages are necessary to support the mitochondrial, enzymatic energy-producing reactions.

In most instances the female and preadolescent male athletes are iron deficient. Such a deficiency is a potential threat to fully realizing one's potential maximal-aerobic power. Since the major role of iron in the body is carrying oxygen, an iron deficiency could seriously affect both the energy producing process during cycling as well as the recovery processes.

Iron is normally stored in the bone marrow, liver, and spleen. With hard training and competition there may be a greater than normal need for iron. This need appears to be especially evident during the early stages of training. There appears to be a need to insure an adequate iron intake in the diets of young boys and especially in diets of girls and women who participate regularly in strenuous cycling. The iron requirement for girls and women during the menstrual years has been stated to be 18 milligrams daily. A low hemoglobin concentration could limit the oxygen carrying capacity of the blood, thereby not allowing full utilization of cardiac output.

## ASSESSING BODY COMPOSITION

Two methods for determining body composition in common use today are: (1) selected anthropometric measures such as skinfolds, skeletal diameters, and body circumferences; and (2) underwater weighing (hydrostatic method). The use of either method provides a good estimate of the individual's muscle mass and percent of body fat. Of the two methods mentioned, the underwater weighing is the most accurate, but requires special skills and equipment. A more practical way to determine body composition of the cyclist is by the use of skinfold-thickness measures.

Skin calipers are used to measure skinfold thickness and representative sites on the body, for example, the skin and subcutaneous fat overlying the base of the scapula or shoulder blade. The skinfold method is reasonably accurate as a determinate of body fat percentage, since more fat is located subcutaneously than anywhere else in the body. Research supports the contention that skinfold-thickness changes are a relatively sensitive indication of a reduction in body fat.

A number of multiple regression equations for estimating body density or specific gravity from skinfold measurements are available. Using skinfold measurements, the percentage of body fat and lean body mass may be calculated. Age, sex, race, and physical fitness can greatly influence skinfold data. Predictive equations attain maximum accuracy only when they are applied to individuals similar to those from which they were derived. Some of the equations produce fat estimates that are in good agreement with data obtained from underwater weighing while others produce such large errors that their validity is seriously questioned. In general, the body-fat percentage is overestimated in the lean individual and underestimated in the obese. Thus, for research purposes, the use of predictive equations for determining body composition is not acceptable. However, when the objective is not critical experimental research, skinfold equations can provide a good estimate of the percent of fat the cyclist is carrying.

Skinfold measurements are often made using a Harpenden skinfold caliper or a Lange skinfold caliper. The Harpenden caliper may be purchased from Quinton Instruments, Department E46, 2121 Terry Ave., Seattle, Wash. 98121, while the Lange is available from Cambridge Scientific Industries, 101 Virginia Ave., Cambridge, Md. 21613. The Harpenden caliper provides greater accuracy; however, it is more expensive than the Lange caliper.

The two equations of Sloan, both of which compute body density $(D_B)$ from which percent of body fat may be derived, are useful for estimating the body composition of cyclists. Both equations were originally derived from college-age populations. They are practical for testing large groups and require a minimum of mathematical calcualtion.

For the male and female cyclists, the following equations may be used:

Male cyclist $-D_B$ = $1.1043 - (0.001327) X_1 - (0.00131) X_2$
Where  $D_B$  = body density
       $X_1$  = thigh skinfold (mm)
       $X_2$  = subscapula skinfold (mm)
Female cyclist $-D_B$ = $1.0764 - (0.00081) X_1 - (0.00088) X_2$
Where  $D_B$  = body density
       $X_1$  = suprailiac skinfold (mm)
       $X_2$  = tricep skinfold (mm)

From the results of the above equations ($D_B$) the percent of body fat may be computed according to the equation of Brozek, et al: [% fat = $(4.570/D_B - 4.142) \times 100$]. Or, from the equation of Siri [% fat = $(4.950/D_B - 4.500) \times 100$].

Once the percent of body fat has been estimated other useful information may be derived, that is, fat weight, lean body weight (LBW), optimal body weight, and so on. Use of the following formulas will provide information to be used when recommending training programs and diet.

LBW = TBW — (TNW × % fat/100)
Fat weight = TBW × % body fat
*Optimal fat weight = 0.08 × LBW
*Optimal body weight = LBW + optimal fat weight
Where     LBW = lean body weight (lb)
          TBW = Total body weight (lb)

When measuring skinfolds, the recommendations published by the Committee on Nutritional Anthropometry of the Food and Nutrition Board of the National Research Council should be followed. The thigh skinfold is taken at the vertical angle on the anterior aspect of the thigh midway between the superior aspect of the patella and anterior-superior iliac spine while the individual is seated in a chair. The subscapular skinfold is measured just below the inferior angle of the scapula, along the natural fold running at a 45-degree angle inferiorly from the spinal column. Measurement of suprailiac skinfold is taken just above the crest of the ilium. The fold is lifted to follow the natural diagonal line at this point. The tricep skinfold is taken midway between the tip of the acromion process and the tip of the olecranon, with the

---

*Both are computed for 8-percent body fat (0.08). This percent may be changed as recommended or desired.

arm extending alongside the body. The skinfold is picked up between the thumb and index finger being careful not to include any muscle tissue. The calipers are applied about 1 centimeter from the fingers holding the skinfold at a depth about equal to the thickness of the fold. Three measures at each location should be made, using the mean as the skinfold thickness.

Athletes participating in different sports differ in body composition. In those sports where the body weight must be moved, that is, cycling, physique and body composition may to a large extent set the limits for success. A study of Olympic cyclists in such events as road racing, road-team time trial, scratch sprint, and individual pursuit indicated significant homogeneity for body size. In this group of Olympic cyclists the mean height was 174.9 centimeters while the mean weight was 68.9 kilograms. Generally, cyclists tend to be mesomorphic and ectomesomorphic in body type. The mesomorphic body type is characterized as being muscular with dominant, connective tissue and bone structure. The ectomorphic body type is characterized by relatively light musculature and a general body structure depicting a preponderance of mass over surface area.

As part of the anthropolgical study of Olympic cyclists, three skinfold — the triceps, subscapular, and suprailiac — were measured. The sum of the three skinfolds for the total cycling group was $19.1 \pm 3.8$ millimeters for an average skinfold of 6.37 millimeters. For purposes of comparison, the total of three skinfolds were $16.7 \pm 3.8$ millimeters ($\bar{x} = 5.57$ millimeters), $21.3 \pm 5.1$ millimeters ($\bar{x} = 7.10$ millimeters), and $21.8 \pm 5.0$ millimeters ($\bar{x} = 7.27$ millimeters) for Olympic marathoners, female middle-distance runners, and male rowers, respectively.

When discussing body composition and athletic success, the question of cause and effect is always present. Is the individual successful because he or she possesses a specific body composition or has the individual developed in a specific way as a result of training for the sport. Heredity, too, plays a significant role in physique. In the sport of cycling, as well as running, rowing, and gymnastics, the difference in performance between individuals possibly can be explained by the differing amounts of fat and lean body mass. For the cyclist it seems desirable to be as lean as possible yet possess good muscle strength. Because no definitive data on male or female cyclists' body composition are available at this time, we might examine what appears desirable using success as the criteria. Body composition for athletes in those sports where body weight is a factor in performance might serve as a guide.

Female champion gymnasts average 13 percent fat, while long-distance runners have been shown to range from 11.7 to 6 percent fat. Male Olympic marathon runners possess about 7.5 percent body fat. International male nordic skiers have been shown to possess about 8.9% body fat.

Using the above information as guidelines and considering the type of work involved in cycling, it seems reasonable to recommend that the female cyclist possess from 8 to 13-percent body fat and the male cyclist 5 to 8-percent body fat. Such low fat mass not only lessens the weight load to be carried but also a low-fat percentage provides a greater opportunity for body heat disipation and therefore less added stress on the cardiovascular system.

With the above in mind it would seem highly desirable to assess lean body weight and its complement, percentage of body fat, at regular intervals throughout the cyclist's training and racing season. This would allow detection of those cyclists who show a tendency toward the accumulation of excess fat. With such knowledge, corrective measures in training loads or diet could be initiated.

## BIBLIOGRAPHY

Bergstrom, J., L. Hermansen, E. Hultman, and B. Saltin, "Diet, Muscle Glycogen and Physical Performance," *Acta Physiol. Scand., 71:* 140 (1967).

Bergstrom, J., and E. Hultman, "A Study of the Glycogen Metabolism During Exercise in Man," *Scand. J. Clin. Invest., 19:*218-228 (1967).

Brooke, J. D., G. J. Davis, and L. F. Green, "The Effects of Normal and Glucose Syrup Work Diets on the Performance of Racing Cyclists," *J. Sports Med., 15:*257-265 (1975).

Brown, C. H., and J. H. Wilmore, "Physical and Physiological Profiles of Champion Women Long Distance Runners," Paper presented at the American College of Sports Medicine, Canadian Association of Sports Sciences Meeting, Toronto, Canada, 1971.

Brozek, J., et al, "Densitometric Analysis of Body Composition: Revision of Some Quantitative Assumptions," *Ann. N. Y. Acad. Sci., 110:*113-140 (1963).

Costill, D. L., R. Bowers, and W. F. Kammer, "Skinfold Estimates of Body Fat Among Marathon Runners," *Med. Sci. Sports, 2:*93-95 (1970).

Costill, D. L., R. Bowers, G. Branam, and K. Sparks, "Muscle Glycogen Utilization During Prolonged Exercise on Successive Days," *J. Appl. Physiol., 31:*834-838 (1971).

Costill, D. L., K. Sparks, R. Gregor, and C. Turner, "Muscle Glycogen Utilization During Exhaustive Running," *J. Appl. Physiol., 31:* 353-356 (1971).

DeGaray, A. L., L. Levine, and J. E. L. Carter (editors), *Genetic and Anthropological Studies of Olympic Athleses,* Academic Press, New York, 1974.

Hanson, J. S. "Maximal Exercise Performance in Members of the U. S. Nordic Ski Team," *J. Appl. Physiol., 35:*592-595 (1973).

Keys, A. (chairman). "Recommendations Concerning Body Measurements for the Characterization of Nutritional Status," *Human Biol., 28:*111-123 (1956).

Saltin, B., and L. Hermansen, "Glycogen Stores and Prolonged Severe Exercise," *Acta Physiol. Scand., 71:*129-139 (1967).

Sloan, A. W. "Estimation of Body Fat in Young Men," *J. Appl. Physiol., 23:*311-315 (1967).

Sloan, A. W., J. J. Burt, and C. S. Blyth, "Estimation of Body Fat in Young Women." *J. Appl. Physiol., 17:*967-970 (1962).

Williams, C. G., C. H. Wyndham, R. Kok, and J. J. E. Von Rahden. "Effect of Training on Maximum Oxygen Uptake and on Anaerobic Metabolism in Man." *Int. Z. Angew Physiol., 24:*18-23 (1967).

Wilmore, J. H., and A. R. Behnke. "Predictability of Lean Body Weight Through Anthropometric Assessment in College Men," *J. Appl. Physiol., 25:*349-355 (1968).

Yuhasz, M. S. "The Effects of Sports Training on Body Fat in Man With Prediction of Optimal Body Weight." Unpublished doctoral dissertation, University of Illinois, Urbana, 1962.

# SECTION 10
# Age and Sex of the Cyclist

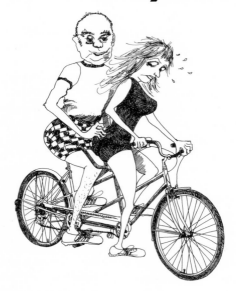

## THE FEMALE CYCLIST

Contemporary widespread increase in physical activity and sport programs for girls and women represents one of the most significant developments in today's sport culture. At one time female participation in competitive sports was discouraged because of societal and cultural stereotypes that considered such participation a departure from the female "traditional role." Consequently, because of the relative newness of female involvement in some sports, such as cycling, many questions concerning the physiological, medical, and psychosocial dimensions of sport participation for the female have been raised.

Competitive cycling for females is relatively new, particularly in the United States. The numbers of girls and women becoming involved in the sport is expanding rapidly for all ages. Unfortunately, for the moment, we have only a partial knowledge of the physiological capability of today's female athlete. Female physiological potential has been estimated by extrapolation from male performances. This practice is unfortunate. Scanty scientific data are available on the female cyclist. Recently there has been some performance data, anatomical and physiological data presented in the scientific literature concerning the female in track and field, swimming, gymnastics, and several team sports. Using knowledge gained from research in other sports an attempt will be made to use that knowledge to benefit the female cyclist.

First, we cannot assume that there are no inherent physiological differences between the sexes. The fact is that there are differences. The extent to which such differences exist and the rationale behind them need clarification.

Research data indicate that the female athlete is stronger and leaner than the average female, has a higher aerobic capacity, and possesses a greater than normal tolerance for lactic acid and oxygen debt. Physiologically, she appears to respond to training much like the male. In comparison with the male athlete, the female possesses a lower body weight-strength ratio and tends to be slightly anemic. However, when expressed in terms of lean body weight, she is equal in strength to the male and equal in aerobic power. Per gram of hemoglobin, the oxygen carrying is equal for both sexes, but a smaller heart volume, smaller pulmonary ventilation, and lower levels of hemoglobin require that for top performance she work at an intensity closer to her maximum $VO_2$ than the male. Muscle fiber composition is similar for both sexes; however, females tend to have smaller slow-/ and fast-twitch fibers. carrying capacity is equal for both sexes, but a smaller heart volume, smaller pulmonary ventilation, and lower levels of hemoglobin require that for top performance she work at an intensity closer to her maximum $\dot{V}O_2$ than the male. Muscle fiber composition is similar for both sexes; however, females tend to have smaller slow- and fast-twitch fibers.

The postpubertal female has less muscle mass per unit of body weight and bone density. In addition, the ratio of adipose tissue to lean body weight varies considerably between the two sexes, to the disadvantage of the female. However, when related to the mass of the active tissue, that is, muscle mass, the potential for strength between the sexes appears similar.

The question often raised is whether a weight-training program will produce a muscular female whose body resembles that of the male. The answer is no. Certain hormones do not allow "muscularization" to occur. In addition, it appears that hypertrophy, muscle cell growth, is not a necessary concomitant with gains in strength. Research evidence indicates that the female does not demonstrate the substantial increases in muscle girth with weight training as does the male. Again, this growth difference is probably due to high androgen levels in the male.

The strength potential of the female is not yet known. In a comparative study, though males had more than doubled the increase in muscle size, their strength gain was slightly less than females. The small bits of scientific evidence suggest that the potential for strength between the sexes appears similar. If in fact strength is not a function of muscle hypertrophy, but rather a neurological phenomenon, there should be no sex differences for potential strength as presently associated with androgen levels.

The use of like training programs for female and male cyclists needs to be considered. Generally the female athlete possesses a larger percent of body fat and a smaller amount of muscle mass than the male athlete. On the average, female endurance athletes possess from 11 to 18 percent fat while male endurance athletes generally possess 8 percent or less body fat. The larger percent of body fat and smaller muscle mass will place a greater work load, that is, cardiovascular stress, on the female than male when engaging in like training protocols. It is essential then that individual rather than common training programs be used. Remember that even though the female cyclist might carry less total body weight, her muscle mass to body weight ratio will be lower than that of the male. This ratio difference becomes quite significant when training or racing where there are hills to climb.

There remains much to learn about the endurance capabilities of female athletes. Women have not had time because of social factors to train long and intensely enough to attain their maximum potential for aerobic power. With more endurance competition available for females, there will be additional incentive to train and maintain high levels of cardiovascular fitness.

The sport of cycling requires rather high levels of both aerobic and anaerobic power. To date, however, little scientific data is available on the aerobic and anaerobic power of successful female cyclists. It is known, however, that national and international class male cyclists possess oxygen-uptake capacities in the range of 55 to 85 milliliters per kilogram per minute. The highest oxygen-uptake capacity recorded for an adult female is 74 milliliters per kilogram per minute. She was a Russian cross-country runner. Values for oxygen uptake as high as 70 and 78 milliliters per kilogram per minute have been reported for 10- and 12-year-old sisters who engaged in cross-country running competition. A study of champion female athletes indicated that, as with the male athlete, oxygen-uptake values are closely related to the aerobic or anaerobic demands of the sport. The central question is: Can the female cyclist reach the level of aerobic and anaerobic power demanded by the sport of cycling? Evidence accumulated from other sports indicates that she can achieve high aerobic and anaerobic power through a scientifically planned conditioning program.

Although there are few training studies involving either young or adult females, the results that have been reported indicate that females respond to the same training stimuli as males, and the training response is similar, for example, greater oxygen-uptake capacity, larger stroke volume, increased hemoglobin, lower resting and working heart rates, increased strength, and so on. This is not to say, of course, that the female will respond to a given training program quantitatively. There is still the question of whether the interaction of frequency, duration, and intensity of training is the same for the female as for the male.

## GYNECOLOGICAL FACTORS

What gynecological factors should the female cyclist be concerned with? Although some research has been conducted in this area, findings are neither consistent nor conclusive. Two frequently asked questions are: (1) What effect do vigorous training routines and intense competition have on the menstrual period? (2) What influence does the menstrual cycle have on athletic performance?

It has been observed that there is great individual variability in duration, amount of flow, and onset of the menstrual cycle. Each of these variables might in some individuals affect their performance in sports. However, when the hypothalamus is chemically stimulated to start its regulation of the menstrual cycle, it does not appear to be influenced by sport participation. For some girls their active competition is in fact concluded before the onset of menarche, for example, young swimmers, while others have begun menstruating before they began sport training and competition.

Before discussing the physiological changes during the menstrual cycle let us first review the phases of the cycle. If fertilization does not occur, the secretion of progesterone is inhibited and the corpus luteum begins to degenerate, which is generally a 10-day process. Estrogen and progesterone levels decrease, and menstruation follows in two to three days. Thus during this menses or dismantling phase there is a reduction of existing estrogen and progesterone in the blood.

Next the follicular or estrogen phase begins where, after the fourth day of menstruation, the blood-estrogen level rises until approximately the fourteenth day or point of ovulation. The last phase is the luteal or progesterone phase. During this phase progesterone is secreted to prepare for fertilization. These cyclic changes in the secretion of estrogen and progesterone influence other functions of the body in addition to the menstrual cycle.

Cyclic changes of estrogen and progesterone influence blood pressure, blood volume, heart rate, vascular tone, body temperature, and electrolyte and water exchange, each of which alone or in combination has the potential of influencing physical performance. The hemoglobin value is highest at the end of the estrogen phase and middle of the progesterone phase. The estrogen or follicular phase occurs about the fourth day of menstruation, and the luteal or progesterone phase occurs about the fifteenth day of the cycle. It has been shown that the red blood cell count and hematocrit and hemoglobin values are all lowest at the onset of menses.

It would appear wise to decrease slightly the intensity of training during the first two days of menstruation. Some reports have indicated performances to be poorest at this time. Although physical performance may not be dramatically altered at the onset of flow, additional stress may be placed on the heart and circulatory and respiratory systems. Blood loss per se during this beginning phase does not appear to affect nor limit aerobic capacity. This is true when iron intake is adequate and anemic low blood volume does not already exist.

High levels of estrogen during the follicular phase are accompanied by retention of sodium and chloride, which results in water retention. The result of fluid retention is a cyclic change in weight, with body weight reaching its maximum value on the second day of menstruation.

Following the maximum weight there is a continual weight loss thereafter for eight days. The additional weight, depending on the amount, could affect cycling performance. In addition, if periodical body composition is determined, it should be scheduled to avoid menstrual cycle influence.

High cyclic levels of estrogen have shown to raise the arousal threshold, increase heart rate, increase cardiac contractile force, increase glucose release from the liver, and decrease kidney output. In addition, during the follicular phase when high levels of estrogen are evident, subtle changes occur in capillary permeability, osmotic pressure, and diffusion; body temperature and metabolism also increase slightly. Whether and to what extent these changes affect cycling performance is not known.

Research reports have indicated that physical performance is best in the postmense or estrogen phase, good in the intermediate or progesterone phase, and poorest in the first few days of menstruation. Based on the various research findings it may be prudent to schedule training sessions and protocol on an individual basis, depending upon phases of the menstrual cycle. For example, training might be intensified during the follicular or estrogen phase, building to maximum intensity from the first day after menses through the fifteenth day.

For most females, heavy training and competitive sports in general have no unfavorable effects on the onset of the menarche. However, females who take part in sports that require much physical effort and endurance, as in cycling, tend to have menstrual disorders more often than other female athletes. Amenorrhea, oligomenorrhea, scanty menstrual flow, or irregular periods occur more often in females participating in those sports requiring strenuous physical exertion over a sustained period of time. In some instances strenuous work during menstruation has resulted in menorrhagia and dysmenorrhea. There is, however, little conclusive evidence that training and competition during menstruation has unfavorable effects on the cycle. Those who have experienced irregular periods or complete amenorrhea during a competitive season have found such irregularities to disappear during the off-season.

Some women competitors claim to have experienced superior performance after the birth of a child. The rationale given is that the strain on the organism produced by pregnancy, a steadily graded effort over a nine-month period, is equivalent to a long-term training period.

No conclusive scientific evidence supports this claim. There is good evidence, however, that females active in sports have shorter labor than the average, and childbirth is no more difficult than for their sedentary counterpart.

The practice of using norethisterone to postpone menstruation because of impending competition is questionable. Toxic effects of the drug on the female as they might affect maximum performance are not known. Neither is there knowledge of the drug effect on the function of the menstrual cycle itself as it affects physical performance.

## THE YOUNG CYCLIST

A discussion concerning age and sport would not be complete without approaching two important questions: What is the proper starting age for cycling specialization? Does very hard physical training have any deleterious effects on the growing child? Both these questions are important, since in cycling hard physical training is engaged in by children to an ever-increasing extent.

During preadolescence there is no essential difference between the work capacity of boys and girls, except that girls reach their maximum work capacity sooner than boys. There are, however, differences between the sexes following puberty. These differences will be discussed later. Although differences exist, it has been established that there is no physiological reason to restrict females from high-intensity aerobic or anaerobic activities.

Some coaches say, "the earlier the better," particularly in the sports of swimming and gymnastics, suggesting the age of six years. Others set the starting age of 16 years in the sport of weight lifting. Training studies suggest there exists a "critical period" for the development of maximum oxygen-uptake capacity or aerobic power. There appears to be a plateau for aerobic power, governed by the time at which physical training is begun. Evidence seems to indicate the existence of an upper limit, over which one cannot surpass, even if the physical training is very intense and extended over several years. For example, it has been suggested that if aerobic training begins at 25 years of age, with an oxygen uptake of 51 milliliters per kilogram per minute, the upper limit expected from training is approximately 64 milliliters per kilogram per minute. However, if aerobic training is begun at 10 years of age, the upper limit is in the high 80 milliliters per kilogram per minute. It might very well be that genetic factors as well as the starting age govern aerobic potential. The extent to which each variable affects oxygen-uptake potential has not been identified.

In addition to the physiological implications of early training, the psychological factors involved must be considered. The emotional impact of early systematic training and competition on the child need careful evaluation. Uncorrectable psychological and sociological damage to the young child must be avoided. It is generally agreed that early-age sport specialization is not prudent. A variety of activities is advised. One-sided specialization, intensive training schedules, and heavy training loads might be delayed until the individual is old enough to realize the consequences of such activity.

Physically well-trained children have demonstrated an increase in maximal aerobic power up to 15 percent in six months. This is approximately the same magnitude shown in young male adults for an equal period of time. In general, the training response seen in the central circulation of young children is in good agreement with that observed after training of middle-aged men and women of varying ages. As with adults, training of young girls and boys results in the heart being capable of pumping more blood per stroke (stroke volume) and per minute (minute volume). However, in contrast to the adult, the ability of the working muscle to extract more oxygen from the blood (a-v oxygen difference) following training does not appear in the young child.

Based on research evidence, children and adolescents should be exposed to a limited amount of anaerobic training. Protocols that produce severe oxygen debts should be avoided until after the pubertal phase has passed (after the first months of the fifteenth year for boys and after the seventh month of 13-year-old girls.) The reason for such avoidance is due to the limited powers for fine regulation of the circulatory system that exist in prepubertal children. The content of the rate-limiting enzyme of the glycolytic or anaerobic energy producing system is low in children when compared with adults. Thus steady-state rather than interval training is best for the young child and adolescent. In addition, no final push or hard long sprint should be encouraged at the end of the ride in order to avoid an anaerobic debt.

Children can attain very high levels of maximal aerobic power (endurance). Generally, the training response seen in the central circulation of young children is in good agreement with that observed after training of middle-aged men and women of varying ages. Like adults, training in young children results in the heart being capable of pumping more blood per beat (stroke volume) and per minute (heart volume). In contrast to the adult, however, the ability of the working muscle to extract more oxygen from the blood (a-v oxygen difference) following training does not appear in the young child. After all variables are accounted for, prepubertal boys (6½ to 12 years) appear to improve their aerobic power to a greater extent than in corresponding training of young adults.

During cycling the increased energy demands of work are met by the increased oxygen uptake. The oxygen uptake is related to the exercise intensity and body weight. For the postpubertal male and female, the same work load per kilogram of body weight is relatively lower for the male. This difference is due to the emerging greater strength to body weight ratio of the male. The result is that at a given work load, that is, cycling up hill, the heart rate is higher for the female than male. The relative increased heart rate for the female depletes the oxygen-transport reserve to a greater extent in girls than in boys. Thus the range of anaerobic participation of energy release is reached at a lower work load in girls. This fact has implications for training loads. Equal training loads for the postpubertal female will not result in equal stress. For the prepubertal girl (6½ to 10½), there is essentially no difference in the physiological response to maximum stress when compared to the prepubertal boy.

When considering the aerobic power of children and how it may be enhanced, age appears to be a critical factor. Between and including ages seven to nine years the child does not have the aerobic power to handle his or her weight as seen in the adult. The eight-year-old child, for example, can increase the basal metabolic rate 9.4 times when maximally stressed, whereas a 17-year-old, adolescent possesses the potential for a 13.5 times basal aerobic power. Even if the young child possesses the same or higher maximal oxygen-uptake capacity per kilogram of body weight than a 17-year-old, lower metabolic efficiency will not allow equal aerobic work. In addition, hemoglobin, the oxygen carrying substance in the blood, per kilogram of body weight is approximately 22 percent less in young boys. These facts make it clear that the young child is not physiologically a small adult. Training and competition programs need to be adjusted to the child's growth status. Cycling distances and gear size should be carefully controlled in order to avoid overstressing the skeletal, muscular, and cardiovascular systems of the growing child.

Research indicates that hard physical training during the growing years results in improved maximal oxygen uptake with highly correlated increased dimensions of several components of the oxygen-transporting system. Up till now there has been no indication that hard aerobic training has had any deleterious effects on the growing child. On the contrary, such training appears to have positively influenced the normal development of the child. Obviously, many questions regarding cycling and the child as they pertain to functional growth remain unanswered.

## THE AGING CYCLIST

With the expanded interest in the sport of competitive cycling has come a growing participation of veteran cyclists. In the sport of cycling the veteran is one who is over 40 years of age. Before embarking on a training program the older athlete should heed certain preliminary precautions. An exercise stress test should be experienced prior to training or competition. Such a test performed on a treadmill or bicycle ergometer serves as a diagnostic tool to determine the specific reaction of the cardiovascular system under stress. Once a physician clears an individual for a stress test, a near maximum effort or exertion to the point of contraindicative symptoms should be elicited. It is essential that the person be given a clean bill of health. During a medically supervised test, the individual may be placed in the most unfavorable position possible with the least personal risk. Assuming all is well, the person can then pursue a training and competitive program with a sense of security. Early individual functional evaluation will eliminate the risk of the person unknowingly extending himself or herself beyond a safe limit.

Many physiological functions are affected by the aging process. The functional decrements generally observed with aging are probably a result of a combination of aging, heredity, conditioning, and years of training. The extent to which deterioration takes place for a given period of time appears to be a function of training involvment. Aging itself influences the amount and type of training one might pursue. For the aging veteran cyclist the intensity and duration of training present some special problems. The older body does not respond to the training stimulus as it may have earlier in life.

For some veteran cyclists, competitive involvment is a first-time, serious athletic experience. To a degree, the training response is governed by the age at which training begins. For example, if aerobic training begins during the young adult years, that is, age 25, aerobic capacity may be improved approximately 40 percent or to a value approaching a $\dot{V}O_2$ maximum of 65 millimiters per kiligram per minute. If, however, training is not begun until 50 years of age, an improvement of about 36 percent might be expected, but to a value approaching a $\dot{V}O_2$ maximum of 52 milliliters per kilogram per minute. Although the difference between potential aerobic power is 20 percent for the beginning training ages of 25 years and 50 years, it does not preclude an improved efficiency of greater than 20 percent. We are suggesting that $\dot{V}O_2$ maximum per se cannot be used as a single variable to predict performance potential. Other factors such as ability to utilize aerobic and anaerobic mechanisms, adjustment to varying environmental conditions, and skill and tactics are important variables to consider when predicting performance potential. Still, it cannot be denied that a high $\dot{V}O_2$ maximum is a requirement for top performance in endurance cycling.

Research evidence suggests that between the ages of 25 to 59 years the anaerobic work capacity decreases about 1 percent per year, even though training continues. Likewise, between the ages of 25 to 55 years, a 30-percent decrement has been observed over the 30-year span for aerobic power. In contrast, only a 12-percent decrement in muscle strength takes place during a 30-year span. It appears that there exists a "biologic constant" inherent in the aging process.

Generally aging is characterized by a reduction in the ability to adapt to and recover from physiological stress. Continued training through the aging years appears to maintain a younger functional capacity longer. The point is that the rate of aging may not be altered with training, but that a person may change his or her position on the aging scale relative to the "normal" for a given age.

## THE VETERAN CYCLIST

Little is known concerning the effects of aging upon human cycling performance. The most comprehensive data available on aging and cycling comes from the Veteran's Time Trials Association of England. After amassing average times for veteran cyclists of various ages for distances of 25 and 50 miles, an interesting observation was made. It was observed that with each advancing year over 40 years of age,

Age and Sex of the Cyclist

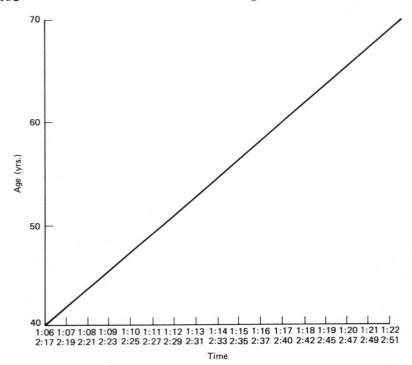

**FIGURE 10.1.** Veteran Time Trials Association of England, times for 25 and 50 miles for the first-class rider.

the cyclist will slow 30 seconds over the 25-mile time trial (Figure 10.1). This falloff in times averages to ½-percent decrement per year. For comparative purposes the effects of aging on swimming times shows a falloff in times of approximately 1 percent per year over ages 25 to 59 years. Likewise, it has been shown that maximal pulmonary ventilation and oxygen uptake approximate a decrement of 1 percent per year during middle age. One might then speculate that these functional changes influence the decrease in physical performance during the middle-age years. It is possible, however, for the aging cyclist to stablize or in some cases reverse the potential performance decrement.

An exception to the above data indicating a falloff in performance of nearly 1 percent per year has been reported for a master distance runner and a cylist. Both of these senior athletes discontinued their training for approximately 38 years when, in their fifth decade, they resumed formal training. In both cases they improved their performances while aging. The cyclist at 71 years of age improved his time for 25 miles by ½-percent over his time at 70 years. Even more amazing is that his 25-mile time of 1:11:16 was equal to a veteran first-class rider, age 50 to 51, which he bettered to 1:07, a time equal to a veteran first-class rider of age 42. From the above data it would appear that increased physical training, even after 50 years of age, has the influence of delaying physiological aging as seen in the average healthy adult.

Veteran cyclists who wish to lower their time-trial time each year despite advancing age will have to increase their training duration and intensity. This implies intensifying training sessions by increasing the pace and shortening rest intervals during interval training.

## BIBLIOGRAPHY

Åstrand, I., P. O. Astrand, and K. Asa. "Reduction in Maximal Oxygen Uptake with Age." *J. Appl. Physiol., 35:*649-654 (1973).

Åstrand, P. O. "The Child in Sport and Physical Activity Physiology." In: *Child in Sport and Physical Activity*, J. G. Albinson and G. M. Andrew (editors). University Park Press, Baltimore, 1976. pp. 19-33.

Åstrand, P. O. "Physical Performance as a Function of Age." *J.A.M.A., 205:*729 (1968).

Åstrand, P. O., B. O. Eriksson, I. Nylander, L. Engstrom, P. Karlberg, B. Saltin, and C. Thoren. "Girl Swimmers With Special Reference to Respiratory and Circulatory Adaptation and Gynaecological and Psychiatric Aspects." *Acta Paediatrica Scand.,* Suppl. *147* (1963).

Brouha, L. "Physiology of Training, INcluding Age and Sex Differences." *J. Sports Med,. 2:*3-11 (1962).

Brown, C. H., J. R. Harrower, and M. F. Deeter. "The Effects of Cross-Country Running on Pre-Adolescent Girls." *Med. Sci. Sports, 4:*1-5 (1972).

Brown C. H., and J. H. Wilmore. "Physical and Physiological Profiles of Champion Women Long Distance Runners." Paper presented at the American College of Sports Medicine, Canadian Association of Sports Sciences Meeting, Toronto, Canada, 1971.

Chapman, E. A. "Cardiovascular Adaptation of the Female Intercollegiate Athlete." Women and Sports Conference Proceedings, Western Illinois University, 1973, pp. 170-184.

Dehn, M. M., and R. A. Bruce. "Longitudinal Variations in Maximal Oxygen Intake With Age and Activity." *J. Appl. Physiol., 33:*

805-807 (1972).

Dobeln, W. V., and B. O. Eriksson. "Physical Training, Growth and Maximal Oxygen Uptake of Boys Aged 11-13 Years." In: *Pediatric Work Physiology*, O. Bar-Or (editor). Proceedings of the Fourth International Symposium, Tel-Aviv, Technodaf, 1972, pp. 93-108.

Eriksson, B. O. "Cardiac Output During Exercise in Pubertal Boys." *Acta Paedia. Scand.*, Suppl. *217:*53-55 (1971).

Eriksson, B. O., "The Child in Sport and Physical Activity–Medical Aspects." In: *Child in Sport and Physical Activity*, J. G. Albinson and G. M. Andrews (editors). University Park Press, Baltimore, 1976. pp. 43-65.

Garlick, M. A., and E. M. Bernauer. "Exercise During the Menstrual Cycle: Variations in Physiological Baselines." *Res. Quart., 39:* 533-542 (1968).

Karlsson, J., et al. *Energikraven Vid Lopning*, Idrottsfysiologi Rapport Nr. 4 (Fourth Edition). Framtiden/Trygg-Flygia, Stockholm. 1970.

Kilbom, A "Physical Training in Women." *Scand. J. Clin. Invest.*, Suppl. *119, 28:*1-34 (1971).

Plowman, S. "Physiological Characteristics of Female Athletes." *Res. Quart., 45:*349-362 (1974).

Pollock, M. L., H. S. Miller, and J. Wilmore. "Physiological Characteristics of Champion American Track Athletes 40 to 75 Years of Age." *Geron., 29:*645-649 (1974).

Rahe, R. H., and R. J. Arthur. "Effects of Aging Upon U. S. Masters Championship Swim Performance." *J. Sports Med., 14:*21-25 (1974).

Rahe, R. H., and R. J. Arthur. "Swim Performance Decrement Over Middle Life." *Med. Sci. Sport, 7:*53-58 (1975).

Robinson, M. F., and P. E. Watson. "Day-to-Day Variations in Body-Weight of Young Women." *Brit. J. Nutr,. 19:*225-235 (1965).

Ryan, A. J., L. A. Ballard, Jr., W. F. Berfeld, et al. "Roundtable: Women in Sports–Are the 'Problems' Real?." *Phys. Sports Med., 3:* 49-56 (1975).

Saltin, B., and P. O. Åstrand. "Maximal Oxygen Uptake in Athletes." *J. Appl. Physiol,. 23:*353-358 (1967).

Skinner, J. S. "Age and Performance." In: *Limiting Factors of Physical*

*Performance,* J. Kev (editor). Georg Thieme Publishers, Stuttgart, Germany. 1973. pp. 271-282.

Thoren, C. "Pediatric Work Physiology—Proceedings of the Karolinska Institutet Symposia." *Acta Pediat. Scand.,* Suppl. *217* (1971).

Wells, C. L., and S. M. Horvath. "Heat Stress Responses Related to the Menstrual Cycle." *J. Appl. Physiol., 35:*1-5 (1973).

Wilmore, J. H. "Alterations in Strength, Body Composition and Anthropometric Measurements Consequent to a 10-week Weight Training Program." *Med. Sci. Sports,* 6:133-138 (1974).

Wilmore, J. H., and P. O. Sigerseth. "Physical Work Capacity of Young Girls, 7-13 Years of Age." *J. Appl. Physiol., 22:*923-928 (1967).

# SECTION 11
# Cycling in the Elements

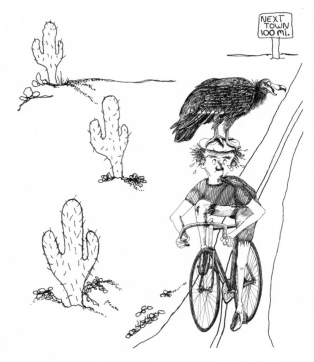

In order to maintain physical work, heat gain must eventually be balanced by heat loss and vice versa. During hard, sustained cycling a marked elevated metabolic state results in heat production that is greater than heat loss. This imbalance may be endured for long durations. However, hot, humid weather conditions can pose particular problems for the unacclimatized cyclist.

Training and racing in hot and humid environments often bring about problems of dehydration, overheating, and fluid replacement. If not met, these physiologic imbalances can exert a negative influence on performance. Proper precycling, during cycling and postcycling measures will serve to greatly reduce the hazards of cycling in the heat.

Fortunately, much of the heat generated by the cycling muscles is lost or transferred to the air surrounding the body by the evaporation of sweat. The constant escape of tissue fluid through the skin plus the action of sweat glands provides surface moisture that when evaporated cools the body. Ambient temperature, air movement, and relative humidity exert great influence on the rate of evaporation. The higher the relative humidity, or water content of the surrounding air, the less effective is heat loss through vaporization. The combined effect of a high ambient temperature and high relative humidity serves to require increased cardiac effort to maintain heat balance. This extra effort detracts from the potential cycling performance.

When the air temperature is higher than body temperature, the effective heat loss mechanism is through evaporation of perspiration. There are other effective avenues of heat exchange such as conduction, convection, and radiation. For the cyclist, heat loss through conduction, that is, making contact with a cooler object, is the least effective avenue for heat exchange. Radiation too is not very effective, since it requires that the surrounding air temperature be less than the body temperature. Conductive heat loss is the process where the blood, which gains metabolic heat, is directed to the superficial vascular beds. The "heated" blood causes the subdermal temperatures to approach body-core temperature. Thus an exchange of heat occurs between the skin surface and the surrounding air. This process is enhanced if the cyclist wears loose-fitting or well-ventilated clothing.

Particularly effective in dissipating body heat are the sweat glands, which are widely distributed over the body surface. They secrete a dilute solution composed chiefly of sodium chloride, urea, and lactic acid. They are controlled by the sympathetic nervous system. When stimulated, the result is dilation of the skin-resistance vessels or arterioles resulting in an increased blood flow to the skin.

The human circulatory system is composed of approximately 70-percent water. Water may be lost at a rate of 1½ to 2 pounds per hour. The vaporization of 1 gram of water removes about 0.6 kilocalories of heat. During cycling performed in a hot, dry environment, sweat secretion may reach values up to 1600 milliliters per hour. The estimated maximum heat loss might be over 900 kilocalories per hour (1600 ml/ hr × 0.58 = 928 kcal/hr). If a cyclist were to ride for four hours under the above conditions, the energy expenditure would represent 3712 kilocalories. This represents a heat loss by vaporization of approximately 12 times normal.

For protection against overheating, the body has a "sweating reservoir" that amounts to approximately 2 percent of body weight. Once this critical level is surpassed, water begins to be removed from the blood plasma. Such removal results in a reduced carrying capacity of the blood for nutrients to the working muscles as well as further heat removal from the body. If preventive measures are not taken to attempt a fluid balance, body temperature will rise leading to heat exhaustion or possible heat stroke.

An elevation of body-core temperature above 40°C (104°F) during hard physical work has been observed in some athletes. However, such high temperatures should be prevented, first, for the safeguard to life and second, to avoid extreme distress. The ingestion of fluids can be beneficial in lowering body-core temperature. In addition to the replacement of fluid volume, the cooling quality of drinking is of value in reducing body temperature.

Among some there is the scientifically unfounded "Spartan" theory that training without liquids "toughens" the athlete. The cyclist who trains hard or races 50 to 80 miles on a hot day needs to practice sound fluid-balance principles. With proper preride, duringride and postride fluid intake there will be a lower body temperature and less stress placed on the cardiovascular system.

When body water is lost by means of sweating, various chemicals are lost as well. For example, sweat is composed of sodium chloride, nitrogeneous urea, glucose, lactic acid, amino acids, and nitrogenous ammonia. When thermal or exercise dehydration occurs, water loss is accompanied by electrolyte losses. Electrolytes are compounds that conduct electric currents in the body. To function properly, they must be in the right fluid compartment in the correct amount. A specific kind and amount of certain electrolytes must be available for normal muscle-cell function. To a degree and in proper balance, electrolytes (sodium chloride, potassium, magnesium) need to be replaced when excessive amounts of water are lost during sweating.

First and foremost, it is important to drink plenty of fluids before, during, and following prolonged heavy training and racing in hot weather. In general, the body's store of electrolytes and the ability of the kidneys to conserve electrolytes during physical exercise will serve to compensate for electrolytes lost in sweat. Those electrolytes that are lost during work can and should be replaced following the training session or race. Replacement may be accomplished through drinking a commercially prepared drink or other substances containing the necessary electrolytes.

Several ready-mixed commercial drinks for fluid, glucose, and electrolyte balance and replacement are available. Most of these commercial drinks have too high an osmotic concentration, which results in the inhibition of fluid absorption. For rapid gastric emptying and absorption, four factors are significant: (1) sugar concentration, (2) electrolyte content, (3) temperature, and (4) volume. A drink containing more than 2-percent sugar, that is, one tablespoon per water bottle, will increase the gastric emptying time or the rate at which water leaves the stomach. Remember our first concern is the rapid replacement of lost water because of sweating. Like sugar, electrolytes too reduce the absorption process. Therefore, if you must purchase a market product, read the content label. If the drink is chilled to between 45 and 55°F, absorption will be enhanced. From a practical standpoint, it is seldom possible to maintain such a fluid temperature while cycling. However, prior to departure and following the ride, it is to one's advantage to chill the drink. Fluid volume up to 600 milliliters (about one water bottle) influences gastric emptying. This does not imply that during the ride one should ingest 600 milliliters of fluid with each drinking interval. However, before departure and following the ride such a volume is suggested.

During prolonged cycling of two to four hours the primary concerns are fluid balance and glucose replacement. With this in mind one of two procedures may be followed. Half an hour prior to departure drink 600 milliliters (one water bottle) of fluid containing 20 to 30 percent glucose. Because of the high-sugar concentration, gastric emptying will be slow; therefore, one should not ingest additional fluid for about 45 minutes. Drinking any sooner will result in fluid buildup in the stomach and an uncomfortable feeling. After the 45-minute delay about two ounces (two hard squeezes of the bottle) may be drunk every 15 minutes. A second procedure begins by drinking approximately 600 milliliters of fluid 10 to 15 minutes before departing. The drink should contain not more than 2 percent sugar, that is, one tablespoon per water bottle. During the ride, about two ounces of a 2 percent sugar solution should be drunk every 15 minutes. Whichever procedure is followed, a well-balanced diet should be adequate for meeting electrolyte needs; however, a replacement drink may be of benefit to some cyclists. Milk contains large amounts of sodium as well as being a good source of potassium. Orange juice too adds potassium as well as fluid to the body. An excellent source of magnesium is spinach. Tomato juice, among other things, is an excellent source of sodium and magnesium.

Dehydration and accompanying electrolyte loss must be avoided if the cyclist expects to function at maximum potential. Chronic dehydration can be avoided by keeping a daily record of nude morning body weight. If weight loss is greater than 3 percent of body weight following a ride and is not regained or body weight progressively decreases, fluid intake should be increased. Thirst cannot be depended upon as an indicator of the need for fluids. It is important to drink plenty of fluids with meals, and in the evening following training and racing in hot weather. To help the cyclist, races as well as training should not be scheduled during the hot hours in summer months and "feeding" rules must be adjusted to meet the conditions of the day.

## EXPOSURE TO COLD

For the serious cyclist, year-round training is essential. During the winter months indoor training on rollers is possible; however, it has limitations. Riding during wet conditions should be avoided for safety. But during cold or hot weather, outdoor training is possible. First and foremost, when training under adverse environmental conditions, is the health and safety of the rider. As weather conditions change during the year, the cyclist is subject to many variables. For example, such variables as low environmental temperature, wind producing a chill factor, heat, and high and low humidity require special adaptive procedures of the rider.

The critical temperature of about 60°F is when most cyclists require additional clothing to their basic cycling shorts and shirt. A basic rule to follow is that the selected clothing should allow the perspiration to vent through. Waterproof nylon shells are not advisable. Wool and cotton are the best materials.

Extra toe protection is necessary when the temperature is about 40° F. Winter cycling shoes with cotton and wool socks seem to meet most conditions. A good pair of leather ski gloves keeps the hands warm. Head and ear protection can be met with a wool ski cap. Ventilated ski goggles provide excellent protection for the eyes.

String-knit, Scandinavian-style underclothing provides excellent absorbing and insulating potential. Generally, several light, wooly layers of clothing are better than one heavy jacket. The several layers allow the cyclist to adjust to the environment as either the body begins to warm or the weather changes. Sweat-dampened clothes do not allow the cyclist to continute to control body temperature effectively. Wet clothing loses its insulation ability and allows heat to escape from the body. Long after the sweat glands have closed down, damp clothing will continue to lose heat by evaporation. The end result is usually a chill. Experience in cycling during cold weather will improve the cyclist's judgment as to selection of clothing.

Under most conditions body heat generated as a result of cycling plus proper clothing will give adequate protection from the cold. However, one must always be alert for possible frostbite in extreme cold weather. Although the air temperature may not be extremely low, the wind-chill index must always be considered (Table 11.1). To figure the wind-chill factor, add wind speed to cycling speed when cycling into the wind.

If prolonged numbness is followed by tingling or "ping" sensation, it is a signal for the onset of frostbite. Where frostbite occurs, the area is white and feels hard. Warm the area as soon as possible. For example, place a warm hand on the affected area until feeling returns (warm the hand in armpit or crotch), or immerse the frostbitten area in water a few degrees above body temperature (100 to 118° F).

During exposure to cold the process of convective heat loss from that portion of the body near the skin surface is reversed.. Exposure to cold results in the withdrawing of blood from the skin to deeper body areas. This action interposes a vasoconstriction between the skin and the cold environment, which offers some degree of thermal insulation. Tissue insulation is even greater if there exists some subcutaneous fat layers. Of course, metabolic heat production is important in extending adjustments to cold.

Another protective mechanism against cold is accomplished by the redistribution of stored calories. In this process, which affects primarily the feet and hands, venous blood normally returning through cutaneous channels is shunted by vasomotor adjustments to veins deeper in the extremity. As a result of the closeness of the arteries and veins, warm arterial blood may lose heat by conduction to the corresponding vein carrying cooler blood centrally. Therefore, there is additional heat exchange within the body. The retained thermal energy reduces heat loss to the environment.

**TABLE 11.1.** Windchill temperatures for cycling speed

| AIR TEMPERATURE (F°) Speed mph | 10 | 15 | 20 | 25 | 35 | 45 |
|---|---|---|---|---|---|---|
| 50 | 31 | 33 | 30 | 28 | 24 | 23 |
| 45 | 32 | 27 | 23 | 19 | 16 | 15 |
| 40 | 23 | 20 | 15 | 11 | 7 | 5 |
| 35 | 18 | 12 | 7 | 3 | -2 | -4 |
| 30 | 12 | 3 | -1 | -5 | -13 | -14 |
| 25 | 3 | -4 | -9 | -15 | -20 | -23 |
| 20 | -2 | -8 | -13 | -18 | -23 | -28 |

Chronic exposure to cold results in a progressive change in the manner in which one attempts to maintain thermal stability. As a result of chronic exposure to cold, some individuals appear to increase their heat production without shivering. Cold acclimatization has been demonstrated by individuals who show an alternation in local circulation during cold stress. This protective process results in hands and feet not cooling as deep, and they generally remain warmer than those who have not been exposed to long-term cold. It appears that the cyclist can become to a certain extent acclimatized to the cold by repeated, local cold exposures. There occurs a shift in the sweating threshold, and the shivering threshold is shifted to a lower temperature level. In addition, thermal discomfort is experienced at lower body temperature. Acclimatization appears to result in a shift to a lower level of the thermoregulatory set point.

From the previous discussion it should be clear by now that cyling endurance is to a great extent determined and limited by the metabolic heat load, by the heat loss conditions, and by the heat gain by sun radiation. These factors, alone or combined, tend to increase body temperature. There is some research evidence to support the view that physical endurance may be prolonged by slightly lowering the resting body temperature before the physical effort. However, such a procedure would interfere with the physiological benefits derived from the prerace warm-ups. It appears that heavy endurance training enhances one's ability to acclimatize to a hot environment. The better trained cyclist will most likely perform best in the heat as well as in normal environmental conditions.

## BIBLIOGRAPHY

Baum, E., K. Brück, and H. P. Schwennicke. "Adaptive Modifications in the Thermoregulatory System of Long-Distance Runners. *J. Appl. Physiol., 40*:404-410 (1976).

Costill, D. L., and K. E. Sparks. "Rapid Fluid Replacement Following Thermal Dehydration." *J. Appl. Physiol., 34*:299-303 (1973).

Costill, D. L., and B. Saltin. "Factors Limiting Gastric Emptying During Rest and Exercise." *J. Appl. Physiol., 37*:679-683 (1974).

Costill, D. L., A. Benett, G. Brabam, and D. Eddy. "Glucose Ingestion at Rest and during Prolonged Exercise." *J. Appl. Physiol., 34*: 764-769 (1973).

Costill, D. L., Kammer, and A. Fisher. "Fluid Ingestion During Distance Running." *Arch. Environ. Health, 21*:520-525 (1970).

Fenn., W. O. "The Role of Potassium in the Physiological Processes." *Physiol. Rev., 20*:377-415 (1940).

Folk, G. E., Jr. *Introduction to Environmental Physiology.* Philadelphia, Lea and Febiger, 1966.

Fordtran, J. S., and B. Saltin. "Gastric Emptying and Intestinal Absorption During Prolonged Severe Exercise." *J. Appl. Physiol., 23*:331-335 (1967).

Pugh, L. G. C. E., J. L. Corbett, and R. H. Johnson. "Rectal Temperatures, Weight Losses and Sweat Rate in Marathon Running." *J. Appl. Physiol., 23*:347-352 (1967).

Rochelle, R. H., and S. M. Horvath. "Metabolic Responses to Food and Acute Cold Stress." *J. Appl. Physiol., 27*:710-714 (1969).

Shvartz, E., A. Magazanik, and Z. Glick. "Thermal Responses During Training In a Temperate Climate." *J. Appl. Physiol., 36*:572-576 (1974).

Wyndham, C. H. "The Physiology of Exercise Under Heat Stress."
    *Ann. Rev. Physiol.*, *35*:193-220 (1973).

# SECTION 12
# Should I Be This Stiff?

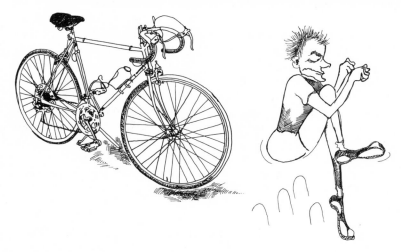

Here we take a brief look at aches and pains—something all cyclists meet at some stage or other. Our intention is to highlight a few areas and not to provide a comprehensive coverage of the gamut of cycling injuries. To do that would require a complete volume by itself and hopefully someone like Creig Hoyt—the medical editor of *Bike World*—can be persuaded to write that book in the near future. Hoyt writes a regular column for *Bike World* in which his experience from seeing many cyclists with a range of medical problems is passed on to the lay reader. If you become a consumer of this column you might find that many people have similar aches and pains to your own and you will certainly find some sound, conservative advice to help alleviate many ailments that bother cyclists.

As a sport, cycling is remarkably free from occupational injuries for which the long-term prognosis is gloomy. This is very different from the tennis players' elbow, the footballers' knee, or the gymnasts' shoulder, which can cause an athlete to give up the sport and also result in an injury that is disabling in the activities of daily living. By far the most serious problem facing cyclists is the danger of falls or collisions and the injuries resulting from subsequent impact. Good equipment and good sense are of course valuable aids, but there are some accidents which, if not unpreventable, could be termed unavoidable. The question then reduces to one of what are the best precautions to take so that when the unavoidable happens, the damage is minimized.

First, in a minor fall, the possibility of serious surface abrasion can be best avoided by having arms and legs covered. When the temperature and humidity are high this kind of advice may clearly lead to heat exhaustion, and each cyclist must find the best solution to the conflicting constraints of risk and cooling for themselves. In many cases the decision might be guided on the basis of road conditions—if you are riding a stretch of road that is likely to be hazardous then keep your shorts packed for another occasion. Certainly, if wearing shorts is motivated by the desire to look like a cyclist, then long pants would be much more sensible.

## THE NEED FOR HEAD PROTECTION

In more serious accidents there is little that can be done about damage to limbs; while it is hardly a comforting thought, breaks and sprains of limb bones and joints are not going to cause permanent damage and may not be much worse than the kind of injuries that result from a fall about the home or office. Head injuries, however, are in a category all of their own. Head injuries from cycling accidents can be every bit as serious as those from motorcycle accidents. It is hard to understand the logic of those motorcyclists who flaunt their disregard and distain for protective headgear, and it is encouraging to see a growing number of cyclists who are wearing helmets on a routine basis. There are quite a variety of models available from bike shops and magazines, ranging from the leather band type seen on racing cyclists—which are probably least effective—to helmets designed for other sports such as canoeing, parachuting, or ice hockey. As yet, since there are no federal or ASTM standards specifically for bicycle helmets, creative manufacturers are attempting to provide their own solution to the specific needs of a cycling helmet.

A complete shell is much more effective than the strips of the racer's helmet; the latter is fine when the impact is on a flat surface but dangerous if there are projections. Some other points to remember when choosing a helmet are lightness, the provision for ventilation, a sturdy chin strap that should be worn at all times, the need to hear once the helmet is in place, and a color that is reflective and useful to improve your visibility to others in addition to its protective function.

## PAIN FROM BAD RIDING POSITION

Many problems in the back, neck, and hand can be caused by a bad riding position, and it is always wise to make some adjustments on the bike as a first step toward therapy. The most common cause for pain is a combination of misadjustments that result in the trunk being inclined much too far forward. In this position several bad things happen: first, the obvious problem of seeing where you are going has to be solved by hyperextension of the neck. This means that the muscles responsible for lifting the head will be subjected to long periods of constant activity that will lead to severe local pain and possible headaches. Second, the trunk also has to be supported against gravity, and this can be done in two ways. Either the muscles of the low back and those on either side of the spine must do more than their share of continuous work, which will again result in pain, or an excessive proportion of the upper body weight can be supported on the hands, and this can lead to a potentially serious neurological disorder than we must consider in more detail.

Although you may not know that you possess this knowledge, you are familiar with at least one place in the body where the ulnar nerve passes close to the surface. Everyone has had the unpleasant experience of banging the inside of the elbow into some object and feeling the pain radiate down the forearm and into the tip of the little finger. What you have done is to compress the ulnar nerve as it passes into the forearm where it will provide some of the wrist and finger muscles with their connection to the brain and spinal cord. In addition, branches of this nerve will connect up with the small sensory organs in the skin, joints, and muscles that continually monitor the state of affairs in the forearm and hand.

There is a second site where the ulnar nerve is again vulnerable, particularly for workers who use their hands a lot and for cyclists and motorcyclists. Figure 12.1 shows what happens to the ulnar nerve during the final part of its course; the particular view shown in the figure is looking down onto the palm of the left hand. The nerve branches into two just as it enters the palm; the dotted region mainly supplies the small muscles of the hand responsible for spreading and drawing

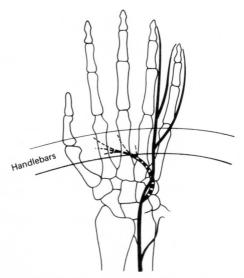

**FIGURE** 12.1. The situation of the ulnar nerve as you look down on the palm of the left hand. The position of the handlebars shows how damage to the nerve can occur by compression.

together the fingers, and drawing the thumb toward the index finger. The portion shown in a solid line is chiefly responsible for sensation in the little finger and the inside of the ring finger.

A typical position of the handlebars in relation to the hand is also shown in the figure, and you can imagine what happens when handlebars and hand are pressed together by the weight of the trunk for long periods, with the additional help of occasional, large forces transmitted through the frame as the front wheel encounters holes and unevenness in the road surface. Fibers of the nerve become compressed, resulting in an inability to transmit impulses in a condition known as compression neuropathy of the ulnar nerve. The symptoms fall into three categories as you would expect from the pattern of innervation just described: (1) you may loose sensation or feel a tingling in the ring and little fingers; (2) you may feel a weakness in the hand; and (3) you may experience both of these symptoms. In the long run, ignoring these warning signs can be very dangerous, since degeneration can occur, leading at worst to a permanent paralysis of the hand. The sad thing about these "worst case" occurrences is that they are very preventable if attention is given to the early warning signs and some changes are made.

The solutions have been well-documented by Hoyt (see reading list at the end of this section) and consist of modifying the bike and changing your hand position on the handlebars frequently during both long and short rides. The most important change to the bike is the use of special, soft rubber handlebar tapes that were developed expressly for this purpose. Since few if any new bikes come equipped with this tape, one of the first things you should do is to strip the thin plastic tape off your bike and go shopping in search of the padded tapes. It will be a small price to pay for vital protection of the hands. Another possible alternative to the tape is to wear padded gloves, but this is generally less practical, particularly in the summer.

Changes that result in better body position include using a combination of shorter handlebar stem and handlebars that do not cause you to be at full stretch. Occasionally the problem may be serious enough for you to consider changing bikes; if this is the case, frames that have more whip in them together with wheels with small-diameter hubs present the most favorable configuration. Whether they have encountered this problem or not, every cyclist should heed the advice of keeping the hands on the move. This can be achieved by holding different regions of the handlebars or brakes and by changing the configurations at the wrists. Above all watch out for the symptoms and, if you do have to visit your doctor, don't forget to tell him that you are a cyclist and don't be bashful about your knowledge of compression neuropathy. You just could be showing your doctor the first case that he or she has ever seen.

## SADDLE SORENESS

There are two major reasons for saddle soreness: a saddle that is at the incorrect height or angle and a saddle-skin interface, which is inadequate. In Section 7 we discussed the correct setting of saddle height. Our measurements have shown that even at the correct saddle height a marker attached to the skin over the hip joint will move up and down through a distance of almost two inches as the cyclist rocks from side to side to shift some of the body weight over the limb that is in its propulsive phase. If the seat is either too high or too low, this rocking of the pelvis will be grossly exaggerated. Depending upon the distances travelled, the kind of material in the seat of the cyclist's pants, and the material used for construction of the saddle, this continual rubbing can cause a variety of problems ranging from minor irritation and redness to seriously infected boils and blisters. The best advice for sufferers seems to be to experiment with seat adjustment, to wear a pair of pants with a special, soft chamois patch in the seat, and to take meticulous precautions to keep skin and pants very clean.

No research has been done on optimal settings for the seat angle, and it must therefore be left for individual experiment with comfort and freedom from soreness being the criterion measures. The same is true for fore and aft position of the saddle, although theories abound concerning the respective merits of different positions. The choice of saddle is a difficult one, too: the plastic saddles will certainly have less friction than their leather counterparts but they will resist the most dedicated efforts to "break them in," that is, to mold them to the contours of the individual.

## KNEE AND ANKLE PAIN

A peculiar thing about joint pain is that one may often have to look at what is happening somewhere else in the body to find the cause of pain at a particular joint. Such is certainly the case at the knee, where the distribution of forces at the foot and ankle can have tremendous influences on knee pathology. Runners and cyclists often suffer from a disorder known as chondromalacia patella in which the articulation between the undersurface of the patella and the femur becomes damaged and cluttered with debris from the damaged joint. In runners, bad foot placement is often blamed, and it does seem that incorrect placement of the feet in the pedals may be the cause of the problem for cyclists, as well as causing strains of capsular ligaments. This is particularly true when the cyclist has cleats on the underside of the shoe which, if incorrectly placed, force the continual use of a potentially damaging foot placement. The way to place cleats is to ride a considerable distance in new cycling shoes until an impression of the pedal is left on the sole of the shoe. The cleat should then be carefully aligned so that when it is in use, the shoe will have the exact orientation of the preferred pattern. Misalignment with the toe pointing in or out is much more critical than incorrect fore and aft placement, although ideally both should be correct.

Good footwear is also a critical element in pain-free cycling. With rubber pedals and on short rides almost anything goes, but the rattrap pedals that are common on ten speeds present problems of their own. Contact between shoe and pedal is limited to the two narrow, metal plates at front and back of the pedal. With a pedal force of 80 pounds-force, and a liberal estimate of 4 x 1/8 in. for the cross section of the supporting surfaces that, because of the serrated edge only make contact along half their length, the pressure on the sole of the foot is in excess of 150 pounds per square inch. With sneakers or other rubber-soled shoes this localized stress will be transmitted to a small area of the foot and severe pain will result from a ride of any distance. Proper cycling shoes have a sole that is reinforced by inserting a rigid plate between the layers of the sole. This effectively distributes the force over a broad area of the foot. Cleats with a large mounting plate are also available, but the reinforced shoes provide a good alternative for the cyclist who feels that cleats are too dangerous because they prevent immediate withdrawl of the foot in emergency. Another factor to watch for is the width of the pedal; some manufacturers make a pedal that seems to be too narrow to accomodate anything but children's shoes. If part of the foot is overhanging, this will increase the stress on the region in contact.

Two frequently blamed culprits for knee pain are high gears and low saddle height, and there is no doubt that both of these factors should be given attention. We have shown earlier that incorrect seat height and a low pedalling rate will both be costly in terms of oxygen uptake, and thus there is a dual reason for attempting to work close to the optimal values. During hill climbing, pedal forces are going to be large regardless of the gear used and, if knee pain persists during hill climbing, medical advice should be sought. It is foolish to dismiss continued joint pain as inevitable. Muscular aches are often trivial and result from the advanced sedentary nature of our "off the bike" lives, but when the warning signals from the joints continue to be received you should pay attention.

## A CAUTIONARY NOTE

Cycling is an activity that can undoubtedly promote good health, and attention to some of the points mentioned in this section can prevent nagging aches and pains from spoiling your enjoyment. A final word of caution is addressed to those who are brand-new to the sport of cycling, particularly those over 35 years of age. There is no reason why you should not be still cycling into your nineties if you take things slowly, but do not forget that such an innocent thing as trying to get to the top of a steep hill without dismounting may take your cardiovascular system up to and beyond its limit. One of the ways a cardiologist will stress test a patient is by stationary bicycle riding with progressively increasing resistance. It is during such controlled tests that cardiac abnormalities are discovered, and routine stress tests may eventually become a part of the preventative medical program of each individual. If you have doubts about your physical condition or if you experience chest pain during exertion on your bike, you must see a doctor. He or she will be able to advise you regarding the kinds of exertion you should undertake and also about how to use your bike as a tool toward progressively better cardiovascular health. Don't think that because you have had a history of heart problems, you will be forbidden from ever riding a bike again. Exercise is a major part of cardiac rehabilitation, and a sensibly used bike is one of the best exercise tools available.

## BIBLIOGRAPHY

Hoyt, Creig S. "Some Unnecessary Pains." *Bike World, 1,* No. 6, 24-26 (1972) and *2,* No. 1, 4-6 (1972).

Hoyt, Creig S. "Numb Hands: A Sequel." *Bike World, 2,* No. 5, 30-31 (1973).

Hoyt, Creig S. "All about Knees." *Bike World, 5,* No. 2, 52-53, (1976).

# Index

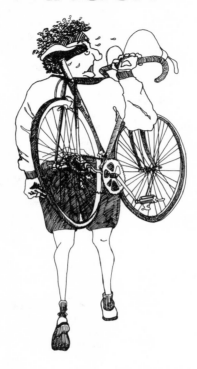